CW00468750

WHO'S IN CHARGE, MY BRAIN OR ME?
(OR MY WIFE...)

Navigating Life With Parkinson's

For Joe & Julie
I'm so happy to have
met you and so grateful
Enjoy your time in Australia
and the read

Claire.

CLAIRE WHITE

First published by Ultimate World Publishing 2023
Copyright © 2023 Claire White

ISBN

Paperback: 978-1-922982-88-9
Ebook: 978-1-922982-89-6

Cover design: Ultimate World Publishing
Layout and typesetting: Ultimate World Publishing
Editor: Rebecca Low

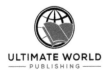

Ultimate World Publishing
Diamond Creek,
Victoria Australia 3089
www.writeabook.com.au

Thank you for contributing to Parkinson's research through the purchase of my book.

DEDICATION

To my husband Errol, whose hot-wired love and action made our wildest cruising dreams possible, jump-starting me. For all of you who understand between the lines, impacting our brains positively, especially our family and friends...thank you.

In memory of Errol's mother, Nan White, and our grandparents for their wisdom, unconditional love, inner strength, and eternal grace.

CONTENTS

INTRODUCTION

Family, pirates, the green flash, fear, last frontiers, dream anchorages, nightmare lightning, hail, rock n' roll, sex, drugs, sharks, crocs, courage, treasure, tragedy, breakdowns, bliss, espionage, the worst storms, the best scenery, flying, favourite living and fishing places, deserted islands, stowaways, pets, provisioning, and Parkinson's, we're asked about them all!

Transitioning from living a joyful, charmed life on the water full-time, mostly anchored far away from marinas, for nearly three decades aboard our monohulls Idlewise and then Restless M, to life on the land is a recognised major life event. It's like a rebirth into the world from a safe womb where we'd been buoyed by a varying level of familiarity, yet encountered daily outside influences, as the weather and scenery changed. Like life, we loved our mothership, and she loved us back.

Voyages loaded with excited anticipation of the great unknown many times took us out of sight of the shore. We remain bold, brave, and fortunate, resiliently weathering life's storms. Not knowing what's around the bend keeps us keenly looking ahead with a positive spin. We just live our amazing, adventurous partnership, now as landlubbers instead of full-time cruisers, and ignore, as much as possible, the fact that Errol also lives with Parkinson's Disease.

My inner compass, set on compassion and trusting my own True North, lives with the rhythms of the tides, cycles of the moon, and seasons of salt and sun on my thirsty skin. Tides of time smoothed us into happier human beings after going through a hell of a rough ride, questioning everything before leaving beautiful Southeast Asia for Australia. My soul's connection to the infinite energy of the Universe is pure magic, removing stress through practicing the eight limbs of yoga, time in nature, social support, setting clear boundaries, and finally with odes of joy, oceans carried us safely home. Voyages, almost one score and ten (30 years) beyond our wildest imaginations and ever-changing horizons became memories, yet our yard was painted by splashes of stunning sunset fires across the water and sky, the moon and stars still shining and shooting for us.

Adaptation and healthy inner reserves of resilience and balance in crisis management, with strategies for safe navigating, are kingpins in weathering stressful storms. Love and connection are lifelines, and we are so grateful for all who give them. When we have a reason to survive life's greatest storms, this strengthens, sustains, and can save us. I kept a laminated family picture for Errol in our survival pack on the boat, thanking God that this photo alone was never needed to keep us alive.

The circle of love and support, inspiring and believing in each other, no matter what is called 'family'. We love our family, no matter what. I choose joy, strength, compassion, harmony, integrity, acceptance, and peace. Inspiration certainly is all around and it's never too late to reassess, get unstuck, courageously hold onto hope, and get back on an even keel, knowing this too shall pass, whatever it is! We got our bounce back, reframed challenges in a positive light, and counted our blessings. It is what it is, yet we all have stories that add colour and flavour, change meanings, and cloud the true light. Experience and criticism can be harsh teachers. Many of our choices give life lessons.

We miss living on the water. Those of you who share that affinity with the ocean will understand. Sure, it's not for everyone, but it's been our life; each loving the sea. There's nothing like the peace the ocean brings to old sea salts. It's beyond understanding. What's important in the end is how well we've loved, lived, and let go. What sparks our joy? Do whatever floats your boat!

Stepping ashore, spring fever came first in the form of a motorhome to keep us moving and exploring. A humble dwelling to call home then grounded us, a new birthday trike bike from me gave Errol freedom and dismount balance, another dream car for himself, surprised me and cheered the landlocked captain, while our boat, still moored nearby, brought added peace. Worldly possessions slowly came ashore, raising the boat's boot line markedly, giving familiarity to our new abode, and adjustment time to trust the process of being land-based near the marina. Furniture materialised, the final piece being my old grand piano, circa 1875 according to our tuner. Getting this ashore is another story. We all struggle with life's challenges, and love makes a house a home, wherever we are.

Safety and practicality had shouted that a small, ground-level dwelling would be wise. Unknowingly, I created our new home borne of singing Christmas carols there. Our Hope Harbour jetty neighbour requested my little group of ukulele-playing midwives and teachers entertain her boss's father, Glaswegian John Brodie, who invited in his neighbours from the over-50s resort-style community just a three or four-minute drive from our marina. I continued viewing many waterfront high-rises as potential homes. Alas, they held plenty of room for isolation, and the clouds and the wind whispered to stay grounded. John later offered his home to us in this delightful community right in our Hope Island neighbourhood, surrounded by trees, a freshwater lake, birds, waterlilies, bountiful kangaroos, a beautiful vista of green all the way to Saltwater Creek, plus all the amenities we could wish for.

Writing became obsessional to share our journey and Parkinson's with packing and unpacking boxes literally in my face. Ironically, I completed a "Living Outside the Box" personal development course, knowing I already live an extraordinary free life! Errol has long understood the advantages of cycling, socialising, and accepting my joy in the slowest of the performing arts: gardening, to replace beachcombing. Familiar hues changed from blues to greens, bringing a bonanza of brilliance between them.

I bless the resting spirits of Hazel Brodie for her beautiful roses and glimpse my long-gone friend Deanne Mitchell's smile in new blooms of bursting colour. Applying gratitude is life-changing, and no matter what changes in our world, when we change our minds to embrace gratitude, there is happiness. Amazingly, the vagus nerve—which influences unconscious body functions like heart rate, blood pressure (BP), and digestion—is activated by simply remembering and re-imagining moments of appreciation. It also forwards these feelings to the brain's pleasure centre.

Psychophysiological unity between the heart, brain, lungs and other body functions is strengthened when treatment includes practicing gratitude.

There is scientific evidence that being in nature, smiling, laughing, receiving healing touch, letting go, practicing forgiveness, showing kindness, expressing gratitude, giving, and experiencing abundance all have profound mental health benefits. It's beneficial to surround ourselves with people who lift our hearts, making us happy. Pleasuring our other senses, such as sight, hearing, and taste, also has numerous health benefits. Colours, waves, music, and chocolate can affect our mood and release endorphins or adrenaline which can calm or excite, altering stress and cognitive function. Knowing what sparks our joy can help us out of a deepening rut. Optimism breeds hope.

"Gratitude makes optimism sustainable." M.J. Fox

Attitude and timing are everything. Life's recognised major stressors came simultaneously: a pandemic, change in country, lifestyle and abode, business sale, family woes, broken leg, hard drugs, and more impulsivity, all causing brain strain! Captain Errol, as an overcomer, avoided frying his wired brain, as smooth, controlled landings ashore reduced Parkinson's killer stress. My mojo returned, packing, unpacking, and living purposely with love, hope, and joy, busting to be resettled.

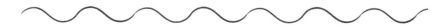

PREFACE

I wrote this book to share our extraordinary cruising story, some health insights, and to give hope. The perspectives of the person living with what sucks, carers, and others, vary. Our brains are soft-wired, modifiable, or neuroplastic. The brain is also brilliant in its capacity to create new connections and restructure existing connections between nerve cells. Brain changes occur when we learn something new or form a new memory. It's constantly adapting and always learning how to learn. Good nutrition is vital, stress is a killer. It inflames the immune system, ferociously firing up nerves. Our brains are hard-wired for love. Love is the answer. It ignites the heart, sending healing to every cell. Focus on enjoying the ride, on the good, and the superpower of happiness comes naturally. Get help if you need it. May you find the way to live your best life.

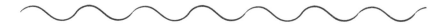

PROLOGUE

by Doctor Barbara Allen

It was about April 2002 that I first met Errol and Claire. He came to me as a patient with headaches and no obvious movement issues at the age of 56. A Darwin neurologist diagnosed him with Parkinson's, which was very low on my radar of possible diagnoses. They invited me and my boyfriend (now husband) aboard Restless M, and we soon joined the large group of people from various walks of life who have the privilege of calling the Whites our friends and have even been on remote Kimberly adventures on Idlewise.

Errol approached his diagnosis as he approaches life—in a practical, positive, and clever way. Having Registered Nurse Claire as a partner was also very helpful. Their journey with Parkinson's has been a combination of research, expert advice, and some cutting-edge decisions. They have maintained their positive and adventurous spirit throughout and now they have replaced the boat with a motorhome. They continue to travel and learn in life and health. This book is a beautifully written account of two interesting, inspirational people, living on a boat AND having Parkinson's. It contains both wonderous and difficult accounts of their ongoing journey.

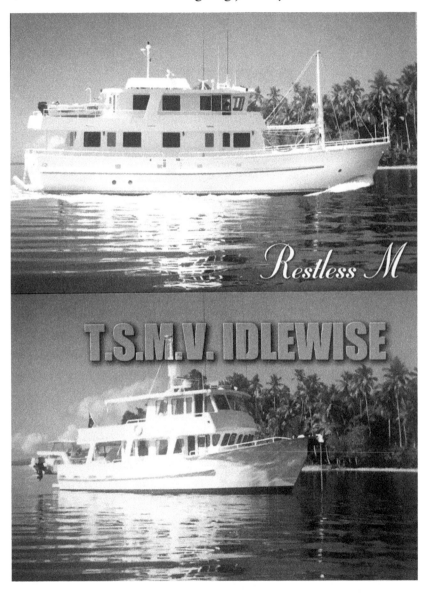

What brings you joy and floats your boat?

CHAPTER 1

LIFE IS BUT A DREAM

I'm a trusting soul, even when my cage is rattled, as I know that tomorrow, the sun will rise again. I aspire to firstly honour my parents, Harold and Margaret Thomson, and my husband Errol with this account of our lives cruising the high seas for eight years pre-diagnosis and over 20 years with Parkinson's.

We make dreams come true through our thoughts, words, actions, habits, and character. The secret to having it all is believing we already do! My faith in abundance and divine timing perfects this. I trust the process, let God or the Universe do the hard work, and magic is sprinkled everywhere.

Seeing the good in all things, I believe, is the key to a charmed life. Of course, with that good come life's lessons, and trust.

Zig Ziglar wrote, "Success occurs where opportunity meets preparation." Anything else is pure chance.

I've been lucky in life and love. I also believe we make our own luck and our own happiness through preparation and opportunity. My heart feels free and at home.

BACK UP...ME HEARTIES FOR A REVERSE SEA CHANGE!

⚓ We're embarking on a new journey, so relax and enjoy the ride! Having written the ship's daily detailed log for years, describing the visible, without adding my emotions overtly is a habit. I bare and share, sometimes too much for some! Perhaps that's my act, as the devil is in the details. I'm happy in the skin I'm in.

My parents taught me that anything is possible, and to go that little bit extra. The difference between ordinary and extraordinary is that little bit EXTRA. Sometimes, I've gone overboard! Writing this book, I've listened to the little voices in my head. I really hope they don't bother you! There's the ✚ nurse's voice, the ⚓ first mate's voice, and of course the ♥ wife's voice. As Errol's greatest advocate, there's his voice too. I'm selective!

I was a nurse and a wife before officially becoming first mate. Sometimes, my own internal captain's voice gives advice. It's great to be your own captain! There are other voices speaking to me too; the Devil's advocate has always been in my ear, sticking up for the underdog, and surely the Devil has been there himself. Yes! He made me do it! God works in mysterious ways and is always with me. I don't bother him, and he doesn't bother me. Got it?

Ascended masters and relatives are also with me in spirit. "What would my grandmothers advise me to do? What would Christ, Buddha, or Muhammad have done?" I've asked Errol, "What would your mother say?" I'm grateful to all who encourage me to do what our wisest taught us!

Being owner-operators of a large boat is like the responsibility of a dairy farm. Regular checking and attendance are required. Automation makes life easier! Self-sufficiency is the goal. Inverters keep things running, but batteries need recharging twice daily by a generator if not connected to shore or solar power. They can overheat. Power can be interrupted (It's not pretty returning from holidays finding thawed freezers). Water tanks, general maintenance, spares, supplies, and waste, need management. Cleanliness is necessary. We always loved it when God washed the boat for us! The exterior was kept simple, with no varnish, minimal stainless steel to polish, and self-draining decks. Rainwater catchment into tanks is easy. Solar energy is almost free, considering the cost of peace of mind, to keep batteries above 80% charged for longer life. Stability is critical.

Errol recharges his 15-year-life Deep Brain Stimulator (DBS) device's chest battery every three to four days. Solar powers our new home. Will it directly charge his DBS battery in the future? New brain stimulator modulation with remote adjustments for ultimate movement and medication effects, gene therapy and designer neurons known as stem cells are some of the research studies and inventions.

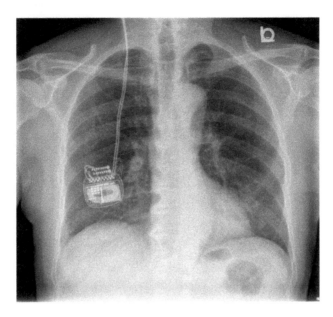

Errol's 15-year battery keeps his computer delivering a very low volt electrical current to his deep brain improving movement and cognitive function especially.

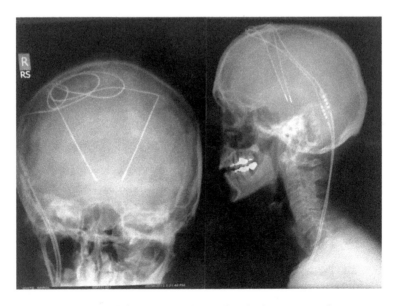

Placement of wires in the Sub Thalamic Nucleus.

One example in Arizona is researchers manipulating damaged or dead adult neurons, reverting them to embryonic stem cells for a wide range of devastating diseases. They have the capability of becoming dopamine-producing neurons forming connections, dispensing dopamine and restoring capacities undermined by Parkinson's destruction of dopaminergic cells. (Dopamine helps transmit brain signals to correctly coordinate movement.) New medications, innovations and breakthroughs for diagnosis and treatment are on the horizon. Thank you for your research contribution. Keeping life simple is a great philosophy. We're planting different seeds, watching for a cure whilst bravely taking new adventures.

HEAD OVER HEELS

✝ I settle my racing heart, having just picked the captain up off the back deck. He also fell two days before when stepping down from our new motor home, misjudging the greater distance since stabilising jacks were down, and landing on his knees. Fortunately, no head injury, nor damage to the new hip was sustained and his mate Ian was there. Just skin off, some blood, and 'kneemoania'.

Nurses are sometimes not as sympathetic to our own because we see cases far worse with greater pain thresholds. Errol is as tough as nails. He left me aboard in peace to write visiting our new house alone. My duty of care doesn't switch off easily. His attitude to wheelie walker use for balance has mellowed as his own shadow and intermittent festinating gait trip him easily. Festination is feet shuffling low and progressively faster, with his body moving forward, more from the shoulders, with an increased likelihood of a subsequent fall forward, especially when he's on his toes. Being a nurse, I can see how lucky he is to have escaped worse injury from the falls he has suffered for so long despite Pilates classes and dancing for strength and balance.

It took discipline for me to stay and focus, knowing I can't wrap him in cotton wool. Some days, his balance is askew. Some days, we ride the wave! Stress worsens everything. He worries most about his immediate family. My detachment and acceptance are critical for good energy. We are intent on finding frayed threads of any silver lining. For harmony, unconditional love, grace and acceptance are keys to restoring balance and inner calm. All parents want their children to be happy together. Sometimes conversational accelerant with a dash of judgement is impulsively thrown on fires and ferociously burns far beyond 'skin deep' to the third-degree. When flushed away with cleansing kindness, valuable truths can soak in, helping heal chronic wounds. Making amends beats tippy-toeing awkwardly around elephants in the room, bringing freedom and forgiveness with no space for regrets. Honesty, integrity, loyalty and kindness are more valuable than gold. Time is more valuable than money. Like the word spoken, spent arrow, and missed opportunity, you cannot get time back. Tick-tock!

Our new neighbours called to say they'd closed our front and garage doors late last night, not knowing Errol had 'bug-bombed' the joint and was just letting it air as per instructions and would return. Seeing cockroaches in the garage had me gasp! Hearing snakes are more active during this breeding time caused a double shudder! We back onto a beautiful reserve. I anticipate hazards, as I am a worst-case scenario thinker, but I also know it's pointless worrying as it only changes our outlook. Forewarned is forearmed.

I'm happy knowing we're in a small and caring community. This is the nature of our lives now. I'll add a lot of catchcries like the cotton wool analogy and whenever I'm a disappointed idealist, Errol says, "It's not a perfect world."

Many people have touched our lives. I aim to share the international language of love, bringing some joy and hope. Through sharing, we become better connected. I have been reminded when writing…"This is simple, this is easy, this is fun!" Thank you, Natasa Denman, for this. I'm a believer! Smiles are contagious!

WARNING BELLS

I'm going to go from ⚓ FIRST MATE mode to ✚ NURSE to WIFE ♥ mode and probably switch from Batsh**-crazy 🦇 White-Witch 🧙 mode to 😇 Angel-Butterfly!

 Buckle up, Buttercup! Variety is the spice of life! The world is full of beauty when hearts are full of love, and while we're loving, we're not judging! When I find myself slipping into judgement, I just need to go and love myself a bit more. Try it!

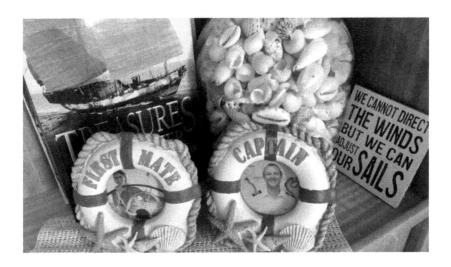

First Mate and Captain

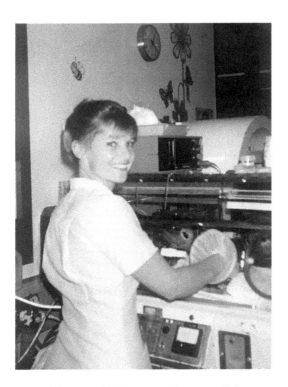

Neonatal Units can be stressful.

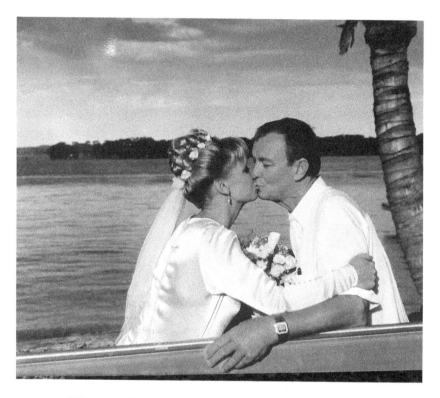

Wearing Grandma's wedding dress and matching cloth shoes, Mum's veil, Dudu's comb, and Josann's hose, we tied the knot, trusting in our future love.

⚓ SORRY ABOUT THE WEATHER!

Everyone asks about our worst storms, pirates, and how many can sleep aboard. My answer to the latter is, that depends on how well they know each other!

Following the weather has been a major component of our voyaging. Yes, we've gone through some terrible storms, both on land and at sea! At times, we were either exhilarated or wished we were somewhere else. Referring to staying in a safe harbour until the weather window opened to head off, Errol would often say, "I would rather be in here wishing I was out there, than out there wishing I was in here!"

Our experiences have helped shape us into who we are now. I love a good cleansing storm, and dancing in the rain! I'm not going to expand on the 30 examples below but will add brief take-homes. Just know our hearts were bounding, bodies in high alert mode, and reliving the memory of how we felt is extraordinary.

Sometimes, life is unpredictable, and solace comes in faith that the sun will rise tomorrow.

Mother Nature sure has dealt us some weather!

*Spectacular lightning too close to Errol's deep brain stimulator frazzles me. Experiencing the flash's powerful smell and white-blue light too close taught respect since Errol can't be defibrillated!

Adrenaline, racing heart, goosebumps, shock, startle, fear—the works! Many of our boating friends have also had direct strikes. This can maim or kill a person, totally disable a vessel, and sink a bank account as electrical repairs are costly. Insurance has become increasingly more expensive against forces of nature and companies will try their hardest to get out of paying.

*Errol's cousin Warren experienced the full might from above, losing a friend to a direct strike through his head when fishing up the Adelaide River in the Northern Territory. He told us it entered through the top and exited through his bottom and no amount of resuscitation changed the outcome. He was burned out. So, when our time is up, it's up!

*Clouds continue amazing us every day in their various forms, reflecting light, playing tricks with our imaginations, dumping energy, snow, ice, and rain, and sending us rainbows. Yes, I have looked at clouds from both sides and searched for the hand of God when memorably skydiving through the rain.

*We've been lucky not to roll over in the 17-foot runabout at Rowley Shoals, WA when bill fishing. Each rolling wave took the body weight of four people to one side of the boat. The risk of capsizing was very present. Being alert to potential disasters can be lifesaving.

*I'm mighty glad I didn't attempt a brag photo pose on that dead, floating massive croc we sidled up to in the Fitzmaurice River N.T. That old fella had everyone fooled. My gut was suspicious that he wasn't dead. Applying caution rather than just jumping right in on the spur of the moment is prudent. Tip: listen to your gut.

*Flooding rain raised the Berkeley River in Western Australia by four metres in the night, adding massive pressure to our anchor's hold, necessitating more anchor chain to avoid being on the rocks downstream. Captain's call was to re-anchor further downstream. Sometimes, doing these things when we don't really feel like it is wise. An extra 6 metres of water had raised the river level by morning. We were glad we'd moved.

*The wind and tide took us sideways onto rocks when amazed by beach-walking elephants in Thailand. Our large surface area added windage, and the pull of the tide, despite fast reaction, made rock scraping unavoidable. Rock bottom is not a fun place to be. Our Indonesian friends Tasya and Wenty will remember this experience and our management.

*Rounding wild Cape Londonderry, WA with wind against tide, the sea stood up horribly. Pitching caused a heavy low fridge dedicated to 14 dozen eggs in cartons to roll right over onto its lid, and amazingly, not one was broken! I'm grateful when things aren't scrambled!

*The outgoing tide has left us high and dry many times, reinforcing that time and tide wait for no man.

*We heard the tide roaring in, then fearfully met a wall of white water a metre high when stuck on the bottom. Our small vessel just floated up over the surf yet could've been swamped. We breathed a sigh of relief. Sometimes, we imagine things could be worse than they are.

*Decks were literally covered by millions of night-flying ants preceding rain, attracted by our whiteness. Crawling around decks with wet wings resembling long skirts appeared laboursome. Come daylight, I noted those not washed overboard through the scuppers into mouths of waiting fish, simply dropped what held them back and wiggled along, seemingly unencumbered in very straight lines around the deck.

I saw how a heavy load can slow and drag us down, and that there are other ways of getting to where we want to go! Going overboard may not always be the best move, growing wings is a miraculous transformation and travelling light has advantages.

*Hail has also covered our decks. BRRRR! Batten the hatches! Our one-wheelhouse perspex hatch didn't crack. Collective sigh!

*Crickets have flown in and found happy places, heard but unseen, like children.

*Birds have sought shelter aboard and left massive calling cards twice their body weight! What can be said about that? Rest up, it'll rain and shoo!

*Travelling with a vigorously flowing tide of about four to five knots, we'd bounced over several shoals in the Bian River, West of Merauke, Indonesia, then ran up hard onto one. With no choice but to wait for the tide, the anchor was deployed, but wouldn't hold, causing us to turn beam to the flooding tide and heel about 20 degrees, the port gunwale awash with mud. We continued seesaw-sliding sideways further over the shoal and came to another halt. The incoming tide and outgoing chain gave hope the anchor would hold, drawing the bow around into the current. It didn't. We remained beam-to (side on), never entirely confident that Idlewise wouldn't capsize.

A combination of shallow water, crocodiles, strong tidal flow, and the potential for our home to flood, with eventual pillaging prior to salvage, was distressing. Lifejackets were on. Errol was convinced the solution was to bring the bow into the current. A second anchor was sought from the lazarette. During location, the ship lurched violently and settled upright again. We were afloat. Hallelujah! Life throws us curve balls that we must sometimes handle, as best we can, with what we have at the time, not distressing ourselves over wild imaginings. We radio forewarned yacht Lara 3 travelling with us. Ahead, they saw our bottom exposed and were horrified.

*In Merauke, South Papua, Indonesia, we set anchor on top of a shipwreck seeing it around us at low tide. Luckily, our ground tackle wasn't fouled.

*We've not entered a massive lake (11 nautical miles in diameter) at the end of Papua's narrow Mamberambo River for fear of getting stuck inside if the lake level dropped!

*We've banged the bottom in the shallow sandy Broadwater of Gold Coast Australia plenty of times and bumped over coral bommies too. Bottom bouncing never feels good. Bless those who help keep our waterways, skyways, and highways accessible and safe.

*A Chinese New Year flaming love lantern landed too close, burning a hole in our timber sponson. Shiver me timbers! They've landed, on yachts, setting folded sails alight. Staying aboard sometimes gives peace of mind.

*Parasailing tourists dropped coral on us from above. The rope of their parasailer speedboat later came too close, caught our mast light, and broke it off. Beware of operators who don't practice Safety First.

*Two F-11s broke the sound barrier with supersonic booms frightening the life out of us at the split-second Errol put Idlewise into gear, resembling a log hitting the propellor. In the Prince Regent River, another two such aircraft wing-waved us low enough to eyeball the pilot (WA) our friends questioning if we knew him and organised this impressive show!

*Coastwatch buzzed us on descent at such speed and close range we worried Nana might have a heart flutter. It warranted discussion. We appreciate border protection from land, sea, and airspace. Drones are a whole new buzz.

24

*Up anchoring in Banda Harbour, Spice Islands, our plow anchor hooked an old, rusty, and very large Admiralty Sea anchor. A buoy was attached to let locals rediscover it. Curiosity had me wondering if it was from an old Dutch trader.

*At the risk of narcosis, I've dived my deepest to 140 feet totally focused on the mission. Errol located and I tied a secure knot on our own set anchor, not our friend's detached ground tackle. Maybe I was narked not recognising our own gear! Buddy Errol couldn't descend more than 120 feet due to ear pain. Our rope on my second dive was initially about three metres short of the surface! Yacht Hope's anchor was abandoned, as time and conditions weren't in our favour. A spare is handy.

*Thousands of Blue Tiger butterflies fluttered by on a breeze, out of sight of land, bound for Shaw Island's flowering Xanthorrhoea Australis (a kind of flax spearhead) in the Whitsunday Islands.

*Hundreds of bats have cooled us with their misty pungent pee-up mangrove-lined creeks. Protecting senses and feeling grateful for paradigm shifts and small mercies is wise.

*We've turned about in fog, anchoring out wide to avoid hungry rats boarding our lines, not trusting our own rudimentary rat stoppers hurriedly fashioned from plastic plates in Jakarta. Avoid the rat race. Let others go first! There are other stories of vermin. We have maintained good practices sufficient to avoid cockroach infestation yet had them fly aboard.

*Just after purchasing Restless M before her refit, we invited our family to join us one evening. It was daylight and massive cockroaches invited themselves out of the woodwork for pizza. I was very happy to strip her right back to the hull.

*We have performed a ceremonious burial at sea of one young stowaway hidden in our runabout while it was under a rural tree for some upholstery work. The runabout was craned back aboard, and the tiny bush rat came inside. The red cover on my iPad sports a chewed reminder that vermin can gnaw through plastic covers on wires and potentially cause an electrical disaster.

*Pods of dolphins racing to us, whales circling and diving under us, birds divebombing or catching a thrown fish frame, feeding sharks, cod and crocs, tuna and rays leaping higher than our aerials, flying fish skimming the surface, dragonfly posing on a fingertip, turtle towing a grandchild, double rainbows over us, sun showers, falling stars and satellites moving, circle round the sun or moon are examples of the awe mother nature offers when time, place and conditions are right.

Whether the weather be fine, or whether the weather be not, whether the weather be cold, or whether the weather be hot, we'll weather the weather, whatever the weather, whether we like it or not!

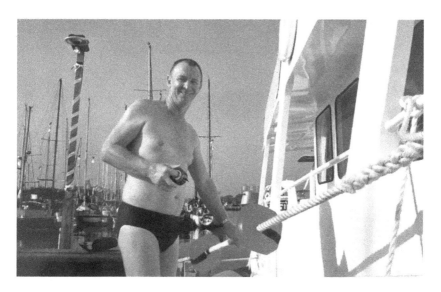

Ancol Marina Jakarta was rampant with rats wanting to come aboard. Leaving the rat race is often the best action.

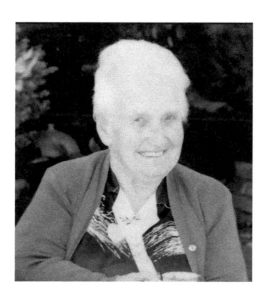

Grandma Mc always said; "Do it while you can!"

CHAPTER 2

THE 7 PS ⚓ SWEET, CHICK, GREEN, SNOW, SPLIT, MUSHY, PEAS, AND QUEUES

Photographing beauty lets the magic linger. With sunrise and sunset, there's often a split second when you can witness perfection. Living in the light adds new dimensions to perceived perfection and many glimpses unfold throughout the day. Yes, we've seen the green flash at sunrise, and at sundown many times. There must be a clear sky with no clouds on the horizon. Polaroid sunglasses help. Yes, we're gratefully in awe of the sun, moon, and stars.

Enthralled by glorious scenery, and water clear enough to see our ground tackle in the deep, we've also encountered mud and some ugliness from sea and land pirates! I'll dine out on them with you later! One question begs, though: why are pirates called pirates? The answer is, of course...because they "Arrrr!"

Getting a Grip: **SAFETY AND STABILITY FIRST**

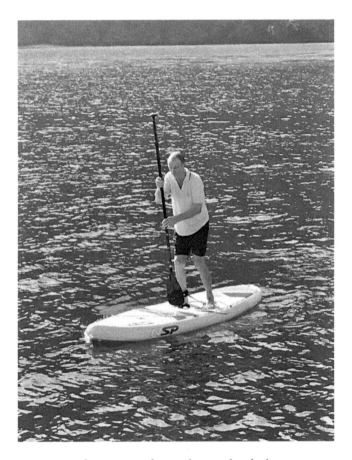

Errol persevered to achieve this balance.

Coupling our sea change to live ashore with acknowledgment of a degenerative neurological disorder, the Safety-First motto is paramount. Balance in life is vital, especially on a boat! Restless M's 80 feet length and stability have given us a safe and comfortable home. Weighing 180 tonnes when fully loaded, her deep draught of 3.3m and heavy belly carries 31,000L of diesel. Yes, it's a big day if saying, "Fill her up!" She has the capacity for holding 20,000L water and 2000L outboard fuel. This weight down low (ballast) increases stability.

She hides about five tonnes of anchoring gear and extra lead ingots forward. She sports rolling chocks angled on each side of the hull, like long tilted surfboards, and is accessorised with paravane stabilisers, deployed only if caught somewhere in rough weather, adding an extra element of stability so we don't spill our drinks! Her ample foredeck boasts a large forward folding mast with a working gantry off a slide-extending boom for loading equipment through the flush-deck hatch. It was lovely sharing this open space, with a large shade boom-tent and room for about seven yoga mats by morning, visiting school children by day, and our flotilla of friends by night.

⚓ Yes, we've rescued stranded sailors, found rafts ashore in remote Australia, pulled a flooding tourist boat off a remote Kimberley rock wall, towed, helped fishermen, relayed emergency radio calls, contacted Australia Maritime Safety Authority (AMSA) when a friend's stricken yacht was caught in extreme weather outside the Great Barrier Reef and non-responsive to arranged HF radio scheduled calls, given repair tools, batteries, spare charts, books, clothing, food, fish and line, flags, ice, fridge, fuel, VHF radios, coffee, coke, beer to grateful Germans, a motorbike, assistance and time. We've found gardening tools in the bush, messages in washed-up glass bottles and searched for another crew's man overboard. There have been tears of sadness and great joy, by us and other families contacted. Daily bread, a kind word, good tea or coffee, and gratefulness can raise spirits more than rum! Alcohol is another story! It's always 5 o'clock happy hour somewhere!

WHO'S IN CHARGE, MY BRAIN OR ME? (OR MY WIFE...)

😇 Kenneth Grahame wrote in *The Wind and the Willows*:

*'Believe me, my young friend, there is **nothing**—absolutely nothing—half so much worth doing as simply messing –about– in—boats, messing...'*

'Look ahead, Rat,' cried the Mole suddenly. It was too late. The boat struck the bank full tilt. The dreamer, the joyous oarsman, lay on his back at the bottom of the boat, his heels in the air.

'—about in boats—or with boats' the Rat went on composedly, picking himself up with a pleasant laugh.

'In or out of 'em, it doesn't matter. Nothing seems to really matter, that's the charm of it. Whether you get away, or whether you don't; whether you arrive at your destination or whether you reach somewhere else, or whether you never get anywhere at all, you are always busy, and you never do anything in particular, and when you've done it there's always something else to do, and you can do it if you like, but you'd much better not...'

Having faith in each other, our safety equipment, and our capabilities, especially when under duress, is also very stabilising. Preparation is key, although there's learning over time called experience. Lives certainly can be in peril at sea. Terra Firma can also be very unforgiving. Some very bumpy glider landings in New Zealand brought this home to me personally. Errol, also being a private pilot, knows well the importance of safety, including routine maintenance and checks. We were lucky to survive a loose fuel line connection in his first Cessna 210 (J.P.L.) evident at about 5,000 feet having departed Padua Park Station near Cunnamulla and emergency landing at St. George,

Queensland (300km away). The aircraft had just undergone our Flying Club's professional routine aircraft maintenance. A natural desire for life preservation and performance confidence is why we requested fresh eyes double-check every system after this hair-raising experience. The outcome could've been fatal. It wasn't our time. Errol returned from a Southport Flying Club's PNG safari very keen to cruise around the magnificent anchorages, seen from above, then we made it happen.

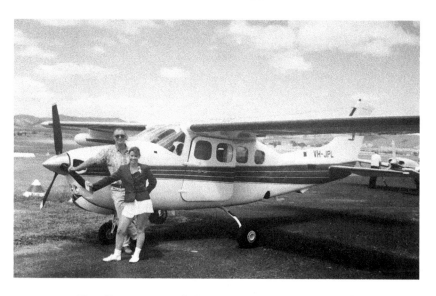

Errol's pressurised Cessna 210 was very smick.

When under pressure, I think Errol is calmer than me, although nursing in the Accident and Emergency Departments really teaches prioritisation and calmness in a crisis. Being able to confront, reassure, help deflect and reduce anxiety calmly and confidently is a skill. I love that he has mostly kept a cool head about him when others are losing theirs! Since DBS, he is more reactive and has experienced panic attacks and learned how to help himself through these, focusing on all senses. I often use the catchphrase, "Worse things happen at sea!" I've also avoided and extinguished his fires.

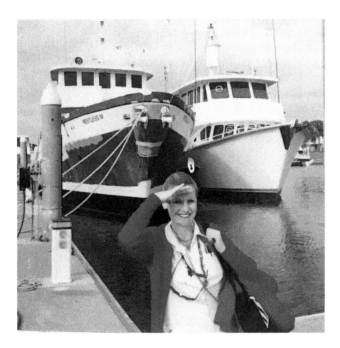

Owning two big boats is usually one too many!

Ah, triumph and tragedy, pleasure and pain, joy and grief, calm and disaster—it's all in a day's nursing!

I've performed minor surgery aboard, removed fishhooks and stitches, organised water ambulances, recommended and accompanied air evacuations, visited many health centres, (and especially, been asked to stay on as a midwife). I've questioned if someone's back required surgical removal from a mattress after excess zzzzzs! We've had some close calls but never—touch wood—had to perform CPR aboard a vessel.

> 😇 *"Peace. It doesn't mean being in a place where there's no noise, trouble, or hard work. It means to be in the midst of those things and still be calm in your heart."*
> —Thich Nhat Hanh

✝ As I write, Errol at 77 years of age has had Parkinson's for over 20 years, with, THANK GOD, a gradual decline in symptoms. Perhaps this is partially attributable to early treatment proactivity and compliance, and he's certainly benefitted from having a nurse at hand 24/7. Everyone's journey is different. The epiphany I had after Errol's brain surgery in 2013 was that to best care for him, I really needed to look after myself first. The carer also needs care.

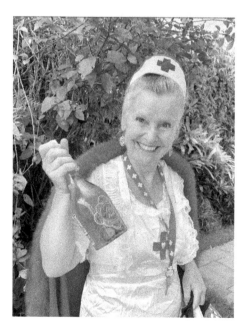

Is it really medicine? Self care is also critical.

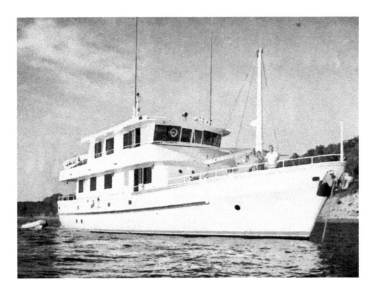

Restless M at Fraser Island before it became known to all as K'gari

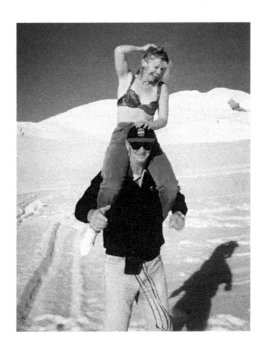

Snow Bunnies on Tasman Glacier, New Zealand.

We've also enjoyed an amazing cruising lifestyle that surpassed any expectation or dream for over 30 years. He was clever, worked smart, and retired at 49, although he states that he never actually retired; he just stopped going to work. Our son-in-law took over the business reins.

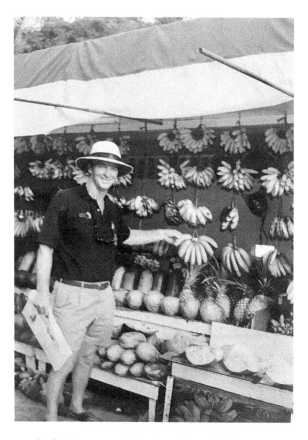

"The Banana Man" as Errol is known.

♥ Moving ashore requires courage. I'm qualified to say Errol is a very lucky man to have such a wonderful wife who loves him and the sea life for this long! This is a big lifestyle change, adjusting and having the best ride possible.

⚓ LIVING SIMPLY

My moving motivation mojo's momentum came in waves! Errol's too as he didn't want to leave our mini ship. Generally, packing up a boat is easier than a house. M.V. Restless M has been our home for 20 years and is a large-volume vessel with lots of storage and lots of belly in the water. In preparation for life ashore, I initially packed up 18 cartons of miscellaneous favourite, joy-sparking things like crystal, family and 21st gifts, photos, shells, extra-musical toys, sasando, conch horn, big gong from Borneo, treasured books, and rocking chair, endeavouring to become more minimalistic.

I have a tendency, like a Bower bird, to collect things, especially shiny things, although I also pride myself on being a rather low-maintenance woman, preferring to reduce, recycle, reuse, reinvent, re-whatever anything, to contribute my little share to looking after our planet and to be thrifty. I also understand that, what you lose on the swings you win on the roundabout, and what you save, you can spend on the dodgems!

Out of sight isn't always out of mind, as what we love stays close to the heart regardless of distance. People and relationships matter more than things. Whatever lies ahead, around us and behind us is minuscule compared to what lies within us.

Kahlil Gibran said, *"You give but little when you give of your possessions it is when you give of yourself that you truly give."* Giving books, pens, clothing, toys, money, and even food has not had the same degree of generosity reward as sharing an experience, especially with children or elders. Sure, gifting money can make a significant difference to somebody's future,

38

especially when used for education or health. Knowing we have made others feel special is the most rewarding. Sing-alongs are a great way to share cheer.

Many friends farewell us with bunches of fresh herbs, flowers, fruitcakes, or produce. It's good to reciprocate in a memorable way. Both sets of my grandparents had fabulous fruit and vegetable gardens and big rambling orchards. Produce has always been gifted, or swapped, even in preserving jars. Sure, I've had many edibles growing aboard, and yes, we've given away a lot of fresh fillets too!

✝ Denial about the need to move off and sell the boat changed in mid-January 2022 when the good captain took a bad fall from standing on a gurney hose. It rolled underfoot, whilst cleaning a sea eagle's splattered picnic remnants, and twice its body weight in poop spread from atop the mast across the foredeck. Landing on his hip fractured Errol's neck of the femur. This was the catalyst for our reverse sea change.

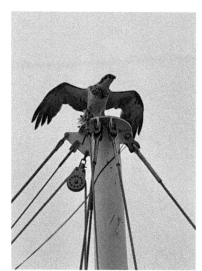

We love bird watching but this eagle was neither welcome nor popular.

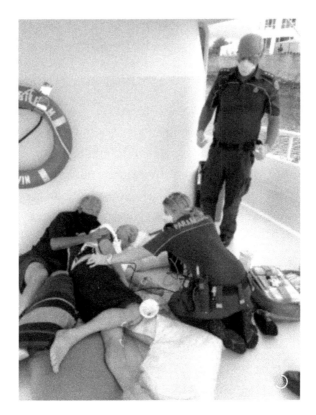

First Responders on the foredeck with Errol

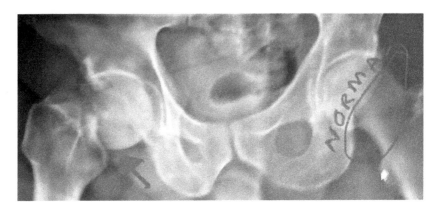

Fractured neck of femur

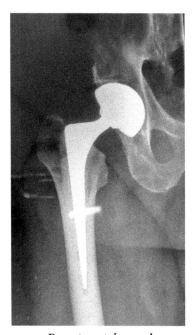

*Repair with total
hip replacement*

I was grateful that we weren't anchored remotely up some Kimberley canyon's backwater, or up the top of Borneo's Kinabatangan River, or outside the Continental Shelf at some deserted island, although the wait we endured for paramedics and then an ambulance made me question if a Heli-rescue via satellite request from those locations could expedite his safety faster.

✝ Hope Island is only 14.2 square kilometres in size. The nearest ambulance station at Runaway Bay is 15 minutes away by road. So, hearing via comms that three ambulances were deployed at the same time to this region was both surprising and frustrating when none arrived after 90 minutes. With a potential raincloud and darkness looming, he needed to transfer to the hospital.

Fortunately, Errol didn't go into shock. I had disposed of unused intravenous equipment and fluids since our return to Australia, after four years cruising Southeast Asia, as it wasn't needed because we were back in civilisation after all!

We appreciate our wonderful Hope Harbour neighbours, of MV 'Last Resort' and 'Investigator' for their assistance. Trained in First Aid, one insisted on being a full body splint, laying alongside Errol to prevent movement and share body heat; Errol

41

is warming to man-hugs! Masks were also now required as the pandemic had reached our local community. Between BP and heart rate checks, I packed some essential items, ensuring Errol had his Parkinson's meds, as he would soon be fasting for surgery.

After a long hour, paramedics arrived and inserted a cannula for intravenous pain relief then, in the next hour, ambulance personnel came, and the magic green pain-relieving whistle (Methoxyflurane) helped. Thank God he only felt the pain when moved. The ball was still in the hip socket but had been rammed right up into it and had broken off at the neck of the femur. Somebody sang, "De thigh bone's connected to de hip bone!" The fire brigade arrived, and with rudimentary splints, Errol was rolled into a big open soft bag with handles, not zippers. Practical yet macabre, we'd carried a zipped mortuary body bag aboard for years. Our supersized chest freezer was back up to accommodate it, as the tropics can be stinking hot. Jokes were made about adding preferred preservative happy hour spirits for the journey. Neither was required, thank goodness! Four fabulous firemen transferred Errol via our starboard side gate, down five white timber stairs, lowering him onto the waiting ambulance stretcher. I cringed for his pain as wheels bumped over every uneven concrete jetty joint.

Errol's next question for the paramedic was, "If I was your relative, which hospital would you take me to?" Without hesitation came the response; a Golden Hip award finalist top-ten in Australia, so there they went. The neighbour of MV 'Wishful Thinking' kindly offered, but I drove myself to the hospital.

Heroes who give the level of care to another human normally given to a family member, or someone else they love, hold the gold standard in my opinion. I believe most nurses do this. Giving care is sacred. Some do go beyond the call of duty. These I call Super Nurse Earth Angels. When we do go the extra mile for someone, it's usually appreciated, making the giver feel good too, it's remembered, and inspires the ripple effect. These days, doing a good turn without the expectation of a return is called 'paying it forward.' Kind and generous souls are everywhere. Total hip replacement surgery was nine hours later.

✝ A good post-operative recovery followed but with some drug-induced delirium and adverse effects on Errol's Parkinson's. He walked well initially post-op, but with opiate pain relief, his balance deteriorated, he slowed, and was more unsteady despite transferring from acute orthopaedic care to an integrated aged care ward three days later. Here, a mix of dementia patients also wandered about, including into his room. Sometimes his neighbour ate his food, and yes, like Goldilocks, sat in his chair, and even attempted to get in his occupied bed!

This neighbour relocated bedside table items to other patients' rooms. I became minimalistic, labelling everything. Sometimes this lost octogenarian would even appear naked at his door, and nurses would whisk her away, chastising her for repeated nakedness. We quietly joked that Errol could still pull the chicks! Of particular concern sadly, were visible open skin breaks especially on her forearms, weeping from constant scratching, and known often unprotected incontinence.

✝ With his brain implant wired to a battery-operated computer in his chest, adjusting to a new artificial hip, and having a large wound, the last complication Errol could afford was cross-infection and prosthetic or implant rejection. Increasing Covid cases were also concerning. Again, I tried to be understanding of the ward situation having empathy. This mix of non-surgical patients went against a lot of my core nursing training, regarding basic hygiene, peace of mind, and privacy, so I advocated for his safety first appealing also for privacy.

He moved beds, 150m away, and was visited by the same mobile neighbour! Soon Errol was well enough for discharge to an assigned rehabilitation hospital with a Parkinson's Disease Warrior Training gym where specific strength and balance exercises in a structured format had proven success. In preparation, some discharge planning was dictated by the consultant as the intern typed, and she read it back aloud from the computer on wheels in Errol's room that oxycodone was to cease due to hallucinations. Hearing this instruction was documented gave me relief.

The admission process went smoothly, the surroundings were newer, and another step closer to home. Unfortunately, at night, Errol was given oxycodone again, resulting in further delirium, causing another four falls with massive consequent bruising as he was having subcutaneous anticoagulant therapy (blood thinners). Seeing him with an allergy alert wristband and preventable bruising added to his discomfort, and to our concern. It was described as most unfortunate in the next hospital family meeting. Thankfully, no dislocation nor damage to his new titanium prosthesis occurred.

For years I'd thought his bone density must be solid with no breaks from falls, but now I became nervous about the potential for more fractures and new hip dislocation. I also worried that he may not regain his full wits. This was particularly hard to think about. Even today, those opioid-induced hallucinations remain very real to Errol, who believed he was in another city during hospitalisation. He admitted he even Google searched his own hospital location for reassurance as everyone he asked, "had it wrong". He hadn't considered himself the common denominator again. Round two of hallucinating had me advocate assertively for a one-on-one or 'special' nurse for his safety.

A decade ago, he was on 'Planet Busy' without opioids post-brain surgery when his implant was over-tuned, stimulating the brain's limbic system and contributing to changeable moods, behaviours, and irritability, (specific regulators are the brain's hippocampus and amygdala) with anxiety taking over and logic becoming panic. Errol became very critical of others and easily provoked. He has always been decent, gentle yet determined and assertive. The captain knows best, makes the decisions, and has semi-joked for years, "There's no democracy on my boat!"

⚓ WORSE THINGS HAPPEN AT SEA!

I can realign a broken nose, have assisted in the relocation of several dislocated shoulders, and have experienced a memorably painful dislocated elbow myself at about age five, yet hips are well beyond my scope. There's a high risk of damage to muscles, nerves, and blood vessels, and it takes a lot of strength to pull even an upper limb back into the joint.

An English Skipper on our rally passage one year to the east in Malaysia, had his artificial hip dislocate whilst simply turning on the bench seat of his inflatable dinghy off the east coast of peninsular Malaysia in the South China Sea. He required 1.5 to 2 hours of evacuation from Tioman Island to the mainland by water ambulance after a failed attempt at joint relocation. This can be a painful, dangerous time and procedure.

"Take a deep breath!" I reminded him repeatedly as respiratory depression occurs with morphine, then oxygen levels drop, and no breathing leads to cardiac arrest. Subsequent re-dislocation caused his withdrawal from the rally. His two crew took his yacht around the tip of Borneo and back to safety.

When cruising, we must be fit, able and prepared for anything. I greatly respect circumnavigators. The second crewman was a Brazilian robotics engineer. Robotics being such a specialised field, I asked if he knew a certain professor of robotics in New Zealand. Yes indeed, they are colleagues! This professor was my very first boyfriend! This small world story reinforces those well-recognised six degrees of separation. The more we share, the more likely these common connections will present.

Crossing the equator by boat earns the title "Shellback". A Golden Shellback is someone who has had the honour of crossing the equator where it dissects the International Date Line in the Pacific Ocean. Rarer still are Emerald Shellbacks having the distinction of crossing the equator at the Prime Meridian in the Gulf of Guinea, West Africa. Paying homage on the equator line to Neptune is a big event. "Pollywogs" have not crossed the equator.

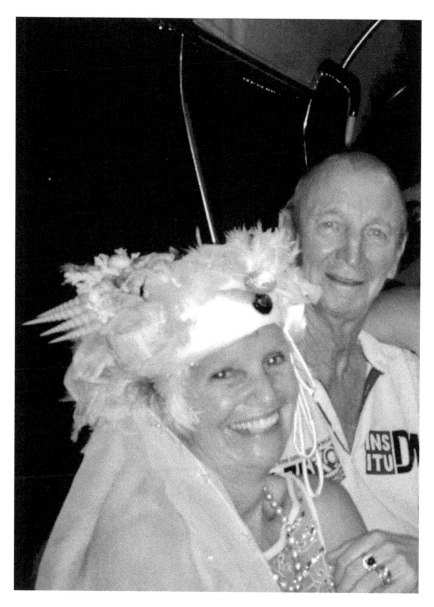

Equator crossing celebrations aboard SY Serica
to keep King Neptune on our side.

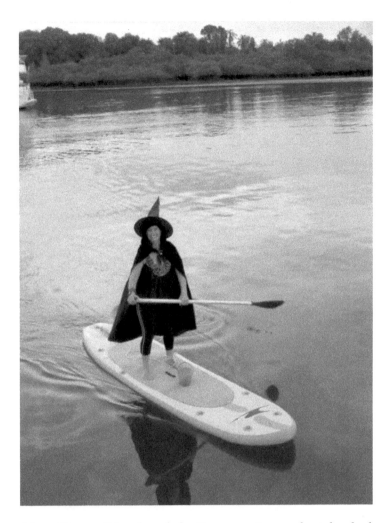

Near Kentor Island and the Equator, I scored tricky slack water for a quick dusk surprise All Saint's Day trip and treat around the anchorage delighting our US citizens.

The 7 Ps are: Prior Preparation and Persistence Prevents Particularly Poor Performance.

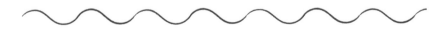

CHAPTER 3

KEEPING BALLS
IN THE AIR

Believing things usually work out for the best, and with Captain Errol in hospital, I had no idea how I would attend the three-day Landmark Forum I'd booked and paid for several months before. It's a transformative learning self-development programme. To maximize benefits, full participation is a requirement. The invitation came from our friend Doctor Barbara Allen, who had originally referred Errol to the neurologist in Darwin in 2002. She has also travelled with her husband and son, both graduates of the programme, to the Kimberley with us several times! On her recommendation, I didn't hesitate to book this three-day transformative forum.

✚ On day two of this course, I was called in by the rehabilitation hospital to settle Errol at 'ugly' o'clock as he was delirious from oxycodone, and they didn't have the 'special' staff to watch him. I was encouraged to be with him primarily because I'm a registered nurse, as well as his wife. Due to the pandemic, visiting was highly restricted. Exemptions were only for birth support or end-of-life circumstances. Staffing was tighter than usual as the pandemic had caused a significant number of nurses to be unable to work.

It's particularly reassuring to know those we love are very well cared for when away from usual surroundings and especially when vulnerable in the hospital. From a giver and receiver's perspective, the gold standard of being nursed well is to be cared for as our own loved one would treat us, and as we would want to be treated. The new 'Golden Rule' is, "Treat others as they would like to be treated."

It was a nerve-racking time, with short-term memory affected by the cortisol released from my own stress. New tech equipment for the course contributed, and techie neighbour PJ was a Godsend. I was able to separate my concerns for Errol's well-being knowing he was in the best place while I attended this zoom course.

It was requested during this Forum that I promise not to take notes to fully participate. This didn't sit well with me, and I've had to deal with that persistently negative issue racketing around repetitively, reinforced by my brain's clever memory shutdown mechanism related to parts of that course. Never had I been requested to not document content from a costly self-development programme!

I now have a much better understanding of being totally present and engaging when somebody else is speaking, listening, and sharing from the heart, without interrupting. My life has always been so full of possibility; knowing all things are possible: opportunity, preparation, action, success, excitement, love, joy, connection, freedom, hope, acceptance, and more.

The Landmark Forum opened my mind to infinite possibilities around the above with extra courage to get my stories out to the world through this book and offer, through our experiences, some hope and help for others, especially those with neurological disorders.

It increased my self-confidence to know that I can do it and be the cause of transformation in others, leaving them moved, inspired, and with more power, freedom, self-expression, and peace of mind. I have freedom from resentment in learning to just love more than judge, forgive more for my own sake, can make decisions without doubting and express my love with a grateful heart. That's peace of mind! Sure, I give credit to my family heritage and experiences for this too.

Similarly, the compelling take-home message from an audiology lecture we attended on our anniversary several months before the fractured hip was this: if you have hearing aids and don't wear them, you're at an increased risk of developing dementia! This is exactly what the audiologist said! It's now proven! He had our attention! There are startling links between hearing loss and cognitive decline.

My understanding is this: when we cannot hear, we use other skills to help comprehension; lip reading, facial expressions, hand, and other body movements to get the gist. This detracts from and interrupts the direct line joining the dots up top, or neuronal transfer. Our amazing brains must soon find other ways to get the message home by strengthening existing connections, forming new connections, or decreasing old, unused pathways.

The brain's neuroplasticity can improve but if we don't use it, we can lose it. With compromises such as hearing loss and translation, it's so busy doing this new circuitry instead of directly comprehending the message in a shorter direct timeframe. As we age, we also tend to 'switch off' when listening gets difficult. We then may miss the conversation's context, answer inappropriately having 'heard' something different, and may even withdraw into our own world of thoughts or nothingness. Communication skills then usually suffer. This powerfully had Errol persevering with wearing and getting used to a device that he did not really like.

Around this time (Dec 2021), Errol also fell in love with a Mazda SUV. It stemmed from a random act of kindness from a stranger who loved hers. We acquired the last white one in stock, each having wheels again. It seems tragic to leave good vehicles uncovered in marina carparks exposed to salt air. Errol was first to ding the newbie driving too close past a parked massive tow bar when distracted by his dashboard of data, bells, and whistles after less than 50 metres of driving on its very collection day. It happens! We had pre-organised insurance yet had to produce emails, texts, and calls to prove it, and endure a routine interview by their fraud assessor. No problem.

Benjamin Franklin said, "Our new Constitution is now established and has an appearance that promises permanency, but in this world, nothing can be said to be certain except death and taxes."

Errol's Australian Business proposals were drafted by others while we were in South East Asia. A wake-up call to get our affairs in order came with these, and as the business was now selling, he keenly wanted his very old will to be updated before, then during hospitalisation. Errol also hadn't paid the current tax bill prior to emergency hospitalisation, and this was a lesson for me to pick up my game and be more involved in our finances. He wanted fairness, to uphold agreements, keeping everyone happy. "No one is born entitled, no work-no pay, inheritance is a gift, not a right, and it's just not a perfect world!" he said.

Expecting people to do what you would do in a situation can lead to disappointment, and may require openness, detachment and acceptance.

My subsequent car accident from behind, during his hospitalisation, was much more extensive than his towbar swipe, wiping out seven passenger side panels taking three months for new doors and parts to arrive from Japan. I was shaken and stirred. Fortunately, no one was injured, and it was still driveable.

THE OPTIMIST CREED Christian D Larsen 1912

PROMISE YOURSELF
To be so strong that nothing
can disturb your peace of mind.
To talk health, happiness, and prosperity
to every person you meet.
To make all your friends feel
that there is something in them
To look at the sunny side of everything
and make your optimism come true.

To think only the best, to work only for the best,
and to expect only the best.
To be just as enthusiastic about the success of others
as you are about your own. To forget the mistakes of the past
and press on to the greater achievements of the future.

To wear a cheerful countenance at all times
and give every living creature you meet a smile.
To give so much time to the improvement of yourself
that you have no time to criticize others.
To be too large for worry, too noble for anger, too strong for fear,
and too happy to permit the presence of trouble.
To think well of yourself and to proclaim this fact to the world,
not in loud words but great deeds.
To live in faith that the whole world is on your side
so long as you are true to the best that is in you.
– Christian D. Larson (1874-1954)

GET YOUR DOSE HERE!

✚ Here's my opportunity for a DOSE boost! There are four feel-good or happy hormones: **Dopamine, Oxytocin, Serotonin, and Endorphins**.

DOPAMINE is a neurotransmitter that's connected to our brain's reward system. It's associated with pleasurable sensations, completing a task, doing self-care activities, eating, celebrating, learning, sex, and memory. It also helps control movement and coordination.

OXYTOCIN is the love hormone that's felt when hugging, playing with a pet, holding hands, giving compliments, in love and sex.

SEROTONIN is known as a mood stabilizer, often felt in running, being exposed to the sun, walking in nature, meditating, swimming, and cycling.

ENDORPHIN is the pain killer found in laughter, comedy, dark chocolate, essential oils, exercise and, you guessed it, sex!

Norepinephrine (AKA Noradrenaline) is produced in nerve endings and is a chemical messenger and hormone. It is part of our body's emergency response system to danger: the fight or flight or acute stress response. It assists in controlling blood pressure (BP) and heart rate. It is made from dopamine, which is produced in the deep brain, the adrenal glands and in the gastrointestinal tract. Dopamine is often referred to as the pleasure chemical or feel-good hormone. People with Parkinson's lose those nerve endings and some of the non-movement features. A sudden drop or irregularity in BP, fatigue, and decreased movement of food through the digestive tract may be attributable to this loss. Errol sometimes has a drop in BP when he stands from a sitting or lying position. Taking time to stand helps equilibrium.

Increasing blood flow improves brain health, memory, focus and cognition. To get our blood moving, exercise is vitally important. Our natural tendency for age-related cognitive decline can be slowed. Nutrients and oxygen in our bloodstream can restore our brain health and by simply increasing the quality of the breath, even over an hour, delivery of nutrients and oxygen is greatly improved via blood vessels to our vital organs. Our blood vessels expand and contract with every heartbeat, allowing our muscles not to be so tight, giving our bones, in my opinion, the best functionality. It makes sense to be more limber. Breathing exercises can be done in a chair, standing up, laying down and when out and about. Tip: keep moving!

One fall in the night from his hospital bed when he couldn't reach the bell and slipped trying to get to the chair meant Errol had to be transferred to another hospital for assessment and to check scans of his head and his new hip. His impulsivity and independence weren't good for him in this instance. Without notification, his Parkinson's medications were ceased completely to investigate the significant drop in BP when standing. I had been monitoring his BP at home and encouraged Errol to drink more as dehydration is a major contributor. Low BP is also a known side effect of his Levodopa and Amantadine medication. Levodopa is used by nerve cells to make dopamine.

Dopamine is a feel-good neurotransmitter. It affects our moods, memory, motivation, and feelings of reward, plus helps regulate body movements, learning, and cognition. Foods that increase dopamine are all animal products, almonds, apples, avocados, bananas, beets, chocolate, and coffee. Protein can affect Levodopa absorption. We can influence our own brain health by 'eating the rainbow', good socialisation, and fuelling our lives with a deep sense of passion, purpose, and meaning. Other ways to increase dopamine levels include good sleep, exercise, music, meditation, sunlight and supplements.

I was glad for investigations and concerned that the drop in BP on standing could also be some other brain or cardiac issue. The hospital neurologist then commenced Madopar, a combination of Levodopa and Benserazide. Errol had trialled it briefly years before without success. As his dopamine levels had decreased, he endured worse symptoms than seen in years.

These included a Parkinsonian mask, causing his face to be like stone, completely emotionless despite smiling on the inside. His saliva glands were highly active, his swallowing was slower and he couldn't help but drool. Blinking almost stopped and his movement became particularly slow, and tiredness affected thought and speech processes. Soon he withdrew and became depressed.

Loss of fine motor skills meant he couldn't even peel a mandarin, cut meat, let alone dress easily, or do up his own buttons and belt. His speech was flat, soft, fast and mumbled. He was also easily emotional and teary. He had difficulty even standing up. You can imagine how we weren't happy with this. All these signs and symptoms led Errol to believe that his Deep Brain Stimulator wasn't working. I assisted him to recharge his DBS battery. It has a fifteen-year lifespan but requires regular recharging, externally via a transducer that just sits on the skin over the small computer positioned just under the skin of his right collarbone (clavicle).

His battery delivers a very low voltage current, via computer to specific areas in his brain (Sub Thalamic Nucleus) and the charge can last for three weeks, apparently. He usually recharges every three to four days to minimize the length of time staying still. We aim to keep it at maximum charge. Previous batteries only had a life span of three to four years, and we planned our travel around surgery replacement, sometimes flying back to Brisbane, Australia. Joking, Errol requested a chest zipper pouch for easier battery changes, doubling as a convenient credit card container!

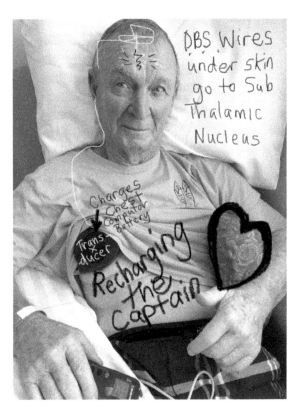

New technology brought Errol a fifteen year rechargeable battery!

Errol re-commenced his usual medications at slightly different times. I was so nervous that he could fall at any moment and spent as much time as possible with him, reassuring him that he would soon improve when the meds were working again. With his dopamine level rising once more, he became much more engaging, his spirit lifted, and his wits stayed sharp. He soon was transferred back to the rehabilitation hospital to continue the physiotherapy sessions.

They really became a fabulous discipline improving his strength and balance which improved his general confidence, giving him a rearing attitude to get home. The team was motivated and integrated with speech and occupational therapists and social workers. He enjoyed watching footy with another patient, Mick, reinforcing the importance of building good social connections in life. This friendship has continued beyond the hospital setting. They both still exercise together.

I also looked for a place for us to live ashore while Errol was an inpatient. After a life at sea, I was sure he would prefer water views.

⚓ The occupational therapist's boat home assessment without Errol present checked out as safe, but the hospital doctor wouldn't sign off on discharge for the jetty nor safety in stepping aboard from our solid stairway from shore to Restless M's heaven on Earth haven. There was no home assessment with him aboard, as it rained the day they planned to return, then they cancelled. It would be prudent for most to stay indoors avoiding wet surfaces.

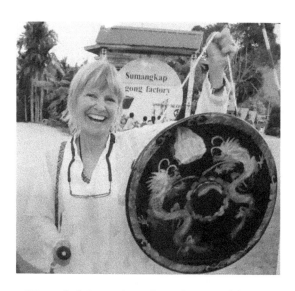

*How did I get this aboard ? Errol knows
I collect musical instruments!*

59

Furthermore, a discharge address of any hotel would have won the doctor's approval, and perhaps held more safety issues for Errol than if he went to his familiar home of some 20 years with grabrails everywhere. How many liveaboards have fallen in the drink right alongside? These perspectives come from landlubbers, not seafarers, but we all know the odd story of a drunken sailor, or of somebody's bicycle going over the side unintentionally of course.

Safety First. It went completely against every nursing fibre in my body to sign the Against Medical Advice form for his release home. He was determined. I read every word aloud to him declaring I would never sign against advice again, nor take the responsibility and the risk as Errol was still impulsive and mostly independent.

I recall one evening parking the car back at the marina, and after taking his Zimmer frame (AKA wheelie-walker) out of the boot, I realised that I needed to straighten up the car, so requested he sit on the walker and wait a moment. He decided to push himself backward whilst seated, then stood up, and fell backward onto the gravelly concrete. Errol is six feet tall. He wasn't knocked out, luckily, but was a bit stunned, said he hadn't seen stars, nor had he hurt himself. His pupils were equal and briskly reactive to my torch light, and he responded appropriately to my orientation questions and commands.

This fall rattled me as the landing was so hard. I wanted to take him to the hospital, then we decided to continue walking home to the boat. Once aboard, I cleaned the gravel from the back of his head, covered and bandaged it, then monitored him neurologically overnight aboard. In retrospect, I should have taken him straight to the hospital. The pressure to be his 24-hour lookout was immense as he didn't see the worst-case scenarios that I did. Brain haemorrhages happen.

We then began house-minding for our family at Currumbin Valley. Two nights are all that Errol had here before three falls and a couple of close calls against large flimsy mirrored sliding wardrobe doors, a glass sliding door and the coffee table to tiles. My concerns going from the boat to the glasshouse also included the flimsy three-sliding glass-doored shower which made up one side wall of the ensuite toilet. My stress levels went up and I was at my wit's end from nervously supervising his unbalanced moves.

My hands went up for help reporting to the physiotherapists, a significant drop in his BP upon standing and an increased frequency of falls. He needed further investigations of strength and balance. I was done being a super nurse, monitoring and doing neurological observations overnight to save him emergency trolly discomfort. Immediate readmission was organised.

Desperate from my worn-out radar, I also contacted myagedcare. com to register us both and receive advice on Aged Care Assessment Team testing and services which couldn't be done whilst hospitalised. They could offer a person to be with him as a companion for one hour once per fortnight, beginning in about a month. I felt it was important for my own well-being to have some time out and continue my weekly arrangement of giving ukulele lessons to a few retired colleagues and friends.

It's important when at the end of one's tether to be able to reach out and ask for help. It's also important to be there for others. I will always be grateful to my friend Helen who was there for me in my 20s when I called from rock bottom.

"I do not understand the mystery of grace—only that it meets us where we are and does not leave us where it found us." Anne Lamott

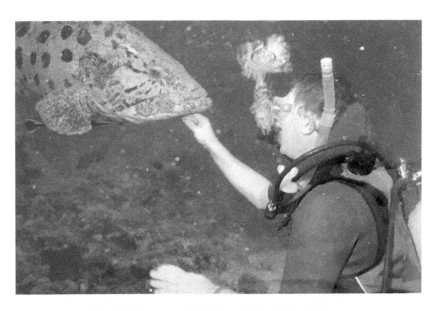

Errol diving on Ribbon #10 with a Potato Cod on Great Barrier Reef

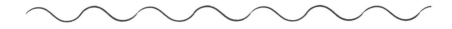

CHAPTER 4

KEEPING OUR SHIP TOGETHER

Postural drop in blood pressure certainly was the cause for a lot of Errol's poor balance. Ironically, a daily dose of fifteen 600mg salt tablets was prescribed to all be dissolved in a 750ml jug of water deliciously salty just for the captain. Daily physio brought improvement. Errol was very compliant when he could see the difference it made to his BP levels.

Cognitive and memory tests were repeated and improved. It does take longer for anaesthetics and opioids to metabolise in older people. A month later when attending the GP for another mental acuity test, the staff laughed saying he was wasting their time, as he was so sharp. Despite this, Errol had to attend three driving lessons and be examined to regain his driver's licence. At a cost of $750 plus the instructor's fees for three sessions, this seemed like a rip-off at the time but initially, there were some cognitive changes affecting short-term memory. Errol came through with flying colours and we understand the importance of safety. The hospital doctor had placed a distance limitation from home on his licence of 20 kilometres and no night driving. We could live with that until wanting to use the new motorhome! The limitation has since been lifted. His speed at serial sevens (counting backwards from 100 in units of seven) always amazes us. He is a numbers man.

After the next month's mental acuity test, we signed our new Wills, Enduring Power of Attorney and Advanced Health Directives before the banana business sold. Errol wanted to ensure before his demise that I would be well looked after. Getting things in order is important for the future.

Discharging back to Currumbin Valley house minding was perfect having changed bedrooms, removing the risk of falling into wardrobe mirrors. The main toilet was safer too with no shower glass wall. Errol used the Zimmer walker during the night. It was like a resort, alas, without the staff! Sometimes we must think outside the box a little and everything falls into place.

At our scheduled six-month appointment in Brisbane, neurologist Professor Silburn was surprised to see Errol using a wheelie-walker and first learned about the hip replacement, reinforcing a lack of medical information sharing. Errol expressed his concerns about the DBS not working and described his inter-hospital transfer fall experience resulting in another hospital neurologist changing all PD meds. The Deep Brain Stimulator device was tested for Errol's reassurance. After some seated simple exercises with thumbs touching fingers at speed, the device was turned off.

As anticipated, Errol temporarily lost his sight. His fine finger exercises weren't performed as well as before and he was not able to stand up from the chair at all. The device was turned on again and he left feeling reassured.

After our friend slipped and fell backward at home, hitting her head, which resulted in a small brain haemorrhage, he took notice and wore his padded helmet again. This intermittently disturbed the functionality of his hearing aids, so if he felt his balance seemed good, the helmet wasn't worn. Then, as his balance improved, he progressed to using a walking stick. In stepping out, we all take a risk.

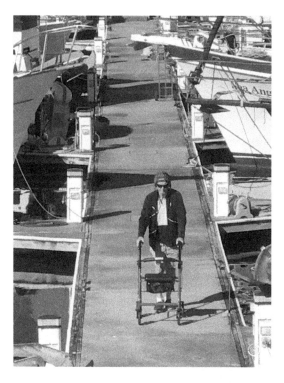

Here is determination, true grit, resilience and a touch of risky defiance.

ERROL'S RUSH OF BLOOD!

It began in Darwin, Northern Territory, Australia when Errol had the first rush of blood one night about potentially owning Restless M over 20 years ago. He didn't want to look back with regret for not having done something.

For four consecutive years, we cruised from Darwin to Ambon during International Yacht races as the communication vessel on TSMV Idlewise, taking twice daily position reports during the race and rally, then cruised back to Australia via various island groups: The Bandas or Spice Islands, The Louisiade Archipelago of volcanic islands fringed by coral reefs in Milne Bay Province Papua New Guinea, Indonesian Kai Islands in the south-eastern Maluku Islands, the Aru group of about 95 low-laying Islands of Eastern Maluku region Indonesia, Merauke in South Papua province Indonesia, Tual and Saumlaki, the Flores Archipelago, Kupang in Timor and Dili in East Timor.

This was a highly adventurous time of exploring new lands and new cultures. After passing Bathurst and Melville Islands and clearing back into Australia, we would either go west and slip across the Joseph Bonaparte Gulf to the Kimberly, or east across the Gulf of Carpentaria and down the coast of Queensland.

Within a few days of being in port, I would return to nursing to sharpen my skills, which got me off the boat and enabled me to also contribute financially to reprovisioning. Being a Darwin-trained midwife who knew and loved the hospital and staff, I was always happy to return, slotting in where needed. Working some graveyard shifts first paved the way. The joy at my return was reciprocated by colleagues. Errol continued essential boat maintenance. There was always a list of jobs waiting. Sometimes, one would come off and another three would be added. It was a full-time job and like many retirees, Errol didn't know how he had found time for work.

RESTLESS M REFIT

⚓ We had a lot of friends with different designed boats that we admired. I loved being able to sit on an open back deck on the main level. Not having that luxury probably did us a favour by keeping us out of the sun for a decade. Errol was excited about taking on the challenge of refitting such a vessel. He had seen her in Townsville years before, knew she was a large-volume vessel and had always admired her lines. He's a big thinker and a real doer.

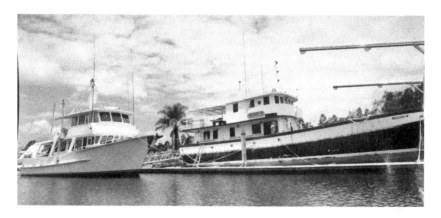

Restless M and Idlewise together

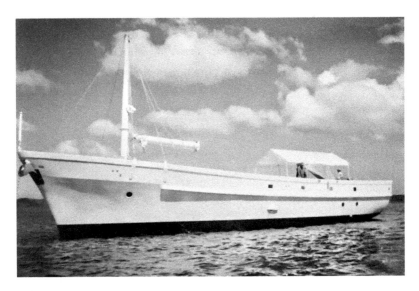

Taking the hull up to meet and marry with the new alloy superstructure in Doughboy Creek Brisbane.

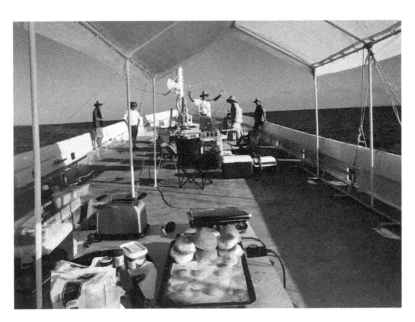

Indeed it was a shady voyage. Errol had the controls duck taped to a workhorse.

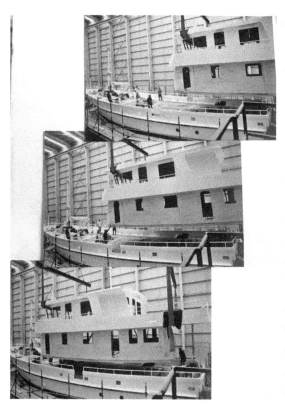

The challenge of refitting an 80-footer was massive. Errol re-engineered her, replacing the GM motor with a slow-revving, straight eight-cylinder Scottish Kelvin Marine engine weighing five tonnes. She served us well and was very economical burning 25L per hour at her most economical cruising speed of 9 knots, including the use of auxiliaries.

Three 10-tonne cranes positioned the new superstructure onto the hull.

We visited the Kelvin and British Polar factory in Glasgow, Scotland and were even given the original papers of the twin engines' flights out to Brisbane, Australia then to Caboolture where they were fitted into the boat built for them: Duchess of the Isles (Dotti). She headed off around the islands of the South Pacific, resting in New Zealand's Milford Sound. We had acquired the first Kelvin in pieces from a friend, John McQuade (RIP). The puzzle to put it back together was another challenge. John and Errol got on well and had a lot in common. He ran dredges out of Southport, had built boats, and like Errol, was very mechanically minded. Years later, after his passing, we bought their motorhome. The first trip 'Maiden Voyage' took us to Angourie, Northern NSW to rendezvous with Indonesian Rally boaties from 2016. Friendships made at sea are also lifelong. We all toasted the McQuades and future travels with the Moët champagne kindly gifted by Lorraine from John's wake.

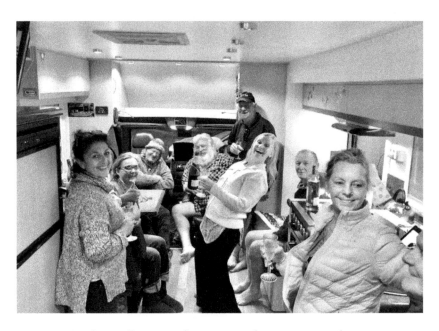

Yacht Rally crew christening the new motorhome.

The first Kelvin was sent up to Caboolture for an overhaul. It was outsourced and unfortunately over-machined, leaking like crazy when dynamo pressure tested. Disappointing! At times, we did wonder if we had bitten off more than we could chew. There was usually some light at the end of the tunnel and Errol's vision remained totally focused. He sourced another Kelvin previously from 'Dotti'.

Idlewise was a perfectly good 65-foot steel monohull and fine for our cruising needs. Errol had always said if Restless M ever became available, he might consider buying her to do her up! I added that I would support him in whatever he decided. We found her tied up at Sanctuary Cove, Gold Coast, Australia. Prior to her return voyage to Australia, she had been impounded by the Indonesian Government in Jakarta over a treasure location dispute, with the authorities wanting their share of the latest Tek Sing treasure from 1999 hauled from the South China Sea with the hunters claiming it was found within international waters. Knowing the $20 Million USD value of the first Nanking Chinese porcelain haul that treasure hunter Mike Hatcher found in the 1980s, his involvement directly in the haul, preparation, and subsequent sales at Christie's auction rooms, the government now wanted their piece of the pie.

With Restless M impounded, it appeared that anything of any value vanished, as she lay apparently neglected at anchor for two years. It's well known that a rush of blood came to Errol one night, ha-ha, and with my encouragement, the deed was done; MV Restless M with all her eyebrow-raising history became ours.

The grandkids all thought she was disgusting, old, rusty, broken, smelly, and cockroach infested. I was very happy to demolish the existing fibreglass-over-plywood house or superstructure and begin completely anew. A lot of solid teak timber came out of her, and Errol's father transformed this in Casino, NSW into well-crafted furniture, including a beautiful coffee table for us. We would both rather not look back with regret for something we haven't done in our lives.

We ran this mini ship, MV Restless M, and before that, TSMV Idlewise, by putting our mark on her, demolishing the old wheelhouse and saloon with a sabre saw, AKA the widow-maker, as he took off the safety guard to get into tight places. Sledgehammers, skill and chainsaws also helped break it up before loading the van and dumping it. I looked hard for any traces of hidden treasure from hunting days. Alas, no gold ingots were found. Captain Mike Hatcher did give us two pieces of ancient Chinese porcelain from one of her hauls; possibly not from the Nanking Cargo, and possibly not dated 1512 A.D. The romance of deep salvage and finding such treasure packaged in tea continues to captivate us.

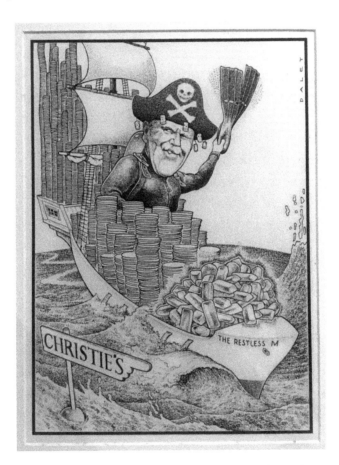

*The Restless M, laden with treasure bound
for Christie's auction rooms, London.*

✝ I loved full-time nursing in the General Medical Assessment Unit (a stabilisation unit for acute cases) at the old Gold Coast Hospital, then devoted myself to midwifery. I nursed in many areas of the new Gold Coast University Hospital to familiarise myself before settling back into midwifery and switched to four days of nursing, and three days per week helping refit Restless M. Here, many stereotypical 'pink' and 'blue' jobs were mine. More gender neutral now, the challenges of adaptation continue, from early chauvinistic conditioning. "When men were men and women were glad of it!" says Errol. Equality is gratefully recognised.

Sourcing, assisting and carrying supplies, including large sheets of marine ply aboard and tidying up tools, power cords and timber shavings was a full-time physical job around my shifts. Wearing gloves also kept my nails clean and I really had a picture of how things were for Errol when he was working in the bank by day and fixing his truck by night B.C. (Before Claire).

Those days were full-on, physically, and mentally satisfying, and we slept like babes. There's nothing like a good day's work, and a clear conscience, to contribute to a fine slumber. A good day's pay sure helps! We were doing this for love which goes around, so the payment has been immeasurable.

Errol was obsessively single-minded. For many hours, his grinder fared the hull in preparation for a new superyacht paint job. The new superstructure by Aluminium Boats Australia was craned on in Doughboy Creek, Brisbane by three 10-tonne ceiling cranes, so the 'coach house' without a coach AKA Wheelhouse without a wheel, was married to the hull with coach screws with us as celebrants! Superyachts Australia continued their painting, and a complete fit-out was done by us with the expert assistance of Shipwrights

Phil, Brennan, and Angus; Rigger Cookie; Engineer Tommy, and so many more, including family from time to time. This was appreciated and took five to six years of our daily dedication.

We fancied giving our forever mate, who wishes to remain anonymous, titles like, "The Foreman", "Project Manager", and later, "Steerage Passenger". Keeping tabs on our progress on multiple visits over coffee or beer and many times, assisting on the big jobs, including the boat's heart operation (Kelvin engine's transplant and hook up), he joined us for the topless voyages to Brisbane for a new superstructure and to Bundaberg, assisting us to limp back prematurely to Gold Coast City Marina's shipyard when the new shaft bearing overheated and then had emergency heart surgery himself on return. His name is engraved on our hearts.

Errol's unwavering tenacity and energy had us all giving our best as he would say, "One day off at this end is another off at the other end of our cruising life." It's not possible here to name everyone who has contributed to building our dreams (you know it, and we are grateful).

Significantly, during the refit, her waterline rose steadily as decades of accumulation were offloaded. Twenty years later, this process was repeated to be shipshape again.

It's said the two best days of a boatie's life are the day of purchase and the day of sale. We know if new owners have half the fun we had, then they're in for a fantastic ride.

So what does M stand for? The best I've heard is Millionaire! M-Multi Mm! RESTLESS M was one of three hand-laid resin ships, her two sister ships, were named either L, N, or O.

HISTORY

She was purpose-built for the ice, in Tampa, Florida, and as a mother ship for a fishing fleet in the Bering Sea and carries 31,000 litres of diesel. Her decks were made wider than usual to accommodate the original owner's wheelchair. I believe she became a floating workshop as a tax deduction for the next owner who pioneered the means of welding cracked cylinder heads known as the Metalock process. We later heard, through the "Ships Nostalgia" site, that the workshop was also a front for drug running in the South Pacific Islands. She subsequently became a salvage vessel operated by United Sub Sea Services. The well-known treasure hunter, Captain Mike Hatcher, then bought her to compliment his searches for treasure and she became his "lucky ship" locating valuable hauls.

Restless M with her all-around and sideband sonar equipment located the Tek Seng haul of ancient Chinese porcelain valued at over $20 million USD. At that time, she also sported a foredeck Hiab crane, a single hyperbaric chamber in the cargo-hold for divers with the bends (decompression sickness) and was registered in London. The second haul of treasure she located was only valued at 10 million USD and was poorer-quality porcelain. Christie's auction rooms then were already flooded with the finer quality ancient Chinese porcelain. Read Hugh Edward's book *Treasures of the Deep* or visit her at work if you google search "*The Lost Fleet of the Guadal Canal.*" Mike Hatcher was a real maritime historian who wanted nothing more than to find a treasure ship laden with gold, silver, and any valuable pieces. He was very keen for us to become future investors.

After the second haul in the South China Sea, the Indonesian government decided they wanted their share of the profits, so impounded the vessel. She then laid at anchor in busy Tanjung Priok Harbour, Jakarta for two years, we believe mostly unattended with no apparent maintenance and although mobile, she soon fell into disrepair.

One of Mike Hatcher's investors said he had 9 million AUD in the project. Despite losing a good five million AUD, he spoke well of Captain Mike Hatcher and was instrumental in bringing the boat back to Australia. At Cooktown, Queensland, she lost her GPS signal and ran aground on a reef suffering rudder loss. A tug towed her into Cairns for repair. She was now registered in Brisbane, sporting this homeport on her transom. We were initially nervous at the prospect of returning to Southeast Asia aboard Restless M for fear that Indonesia may still try impounding her.

We always aim to stay on the straight and narrow and kept Restless M's good name as her fascinating and colourful history already made her a target for the sea gods. It's commonly believed that it's extremely bad luck to change a boat's name, yet I have been sorely tempted to add the letter E. It seemed strangely fitting for Errol with his Parkinson's to have a boat named Restless M.

Her new port of registration became Darwin, where we'd met. With less bureaucratic red tape polluting its waterways, Darwin was also a good base for setting off to God's country, the Kimberley, and to revisit Southeast Asia or cruise back down to family in Queensland, and New Zealand. Whenever crossing the equator, we've marked the occasion memorably to honour and respect the sea god Neptune. We don't want any trouble!

MV Restless M had four multipurpose runabouts and postie-bike, fishing rods galore, my grand piano, a comprehensive wardrobe for entertaining and a collection of musical instruments ideal for impromptu jams. I had to justify having four or five spare ukuleles aboard. Errol stated how ridiculous this was as I could only play one at a time. I just breathed, then slowly explained that each is slightly different and that others can use them, that it's good to have a backup. He knows I have gifted a few ukes and finally, I likened my collection to his fishing rod collection. Silence. Pure gold!

"Wisdom and Knowledge will be the stability of your time and the strength of your salvation." Isaiah 33:6 KJV

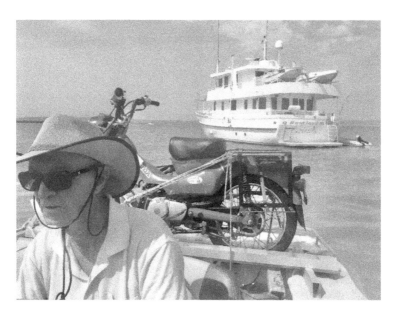

Heading ashore up the muddy Cambridge Gulf to the old port town of Windham.

CHAPTER 5

INSPIRATIONAL PRINCESS SIENA

The Circle of Birth-Life-Death

✝ The word midwife means with woman. Decades ago, whilst practicing midwifery in the delivery ward of the Royal Darwin Hospital, I was allocated to be with an Aboriginal woman from Yirrkala, East Arnhemland. Dedicated flights brought qualifying women into Darwin early for safety.

I expected a shy and frightened woman with little or no family support, but upon entering her room, was surprised by concerto piano music, an incredibly receptive strong woman in labour and noted colourful fabrics, bean bags and a very young Aboriginal girl of about five years old, with a beautiful smile and the whitest teeth. As I introduced myself to the prospective parents, Merrkiyawuy and her husband Will, this young girl had time and the opportunity to check me out.

That day, as air conditioning made my legs cold, I had worn black stockings. I had no idea that this young girl would see me as being half black and white having never in her short tropical life seen anything like pantyhose. It became evident she was puzzled by my skin, so I stretched out the tights at my shin, using my finger and thumb. Her eyeballs nearly fell out to see such amazing, stretchy skin!

Time was well spent whilst waiting for this much-wanted baby's arrival around maternal comfort. I massaged her lower back and her husband took over. When he joked for a massage, I obliged, then an adult daughter joined the peace train. I believe a healing touch is a superpower.

Long awaited baby Siena arrived, named after the town in Italy they loved when travelling with their local band Yothu-Yindi throughout Europe. It's so disappointing when camera batteries are flat, but this momentous day was captured on film as surprisingly I had two cameras in my bag and gave full use of them. Afterward, they encouraged me to share celebratory Moët and sent flowers near my birthday. Of course, I'd taken photos too, had films developed, and forwarded doubles.

On my own birthday eve, I supported another labouring woman from afar with a known foetal death in utero. Yes, midwifery is 99% wonderful and miraculous yet 1% horrendous. Errol had a colourful bucketful of beautiful roses waiting, something small in his pocket and took me out for breakfast. I hadn't mentioned my shift and his proposal closed the circle of birth, death and marriage in one day. My engagement ring, resembling my grandmother's setting, needed resizing.

The jewellery assistants asked how Errol proposed, so I shared that I'm a midwife, and worked the night before his proposal, into my own birthday. They said, "Oh, it must be a wonderful profession bringing life into the world, especially on your own birthday!" I hesitated, then shared that it's mostly miraculously wonderful, adding that my shift didn't have the happy ending of a living baby and that the mother knew this on admission. They looked at each other with understanding that the same young woman had likely chosen with them, a small urn for her baby's ashes the week before. It's a small world. Grief is the price we pay for love.

⚓ Leaving Darwin and NT friends was always a little sad, yet other friends and family welcomed us on the other side, once over the top of Arnhemland and beyond the beautiful Wessel Islands to the East. We anchored off Inverell Bay near The Gove Boat Club, where I paid respects to my old skipper/commodore Bill, reprovisioned and re-joined our special friends from the aboriginal community of Yirrkala year after year. In the circle of life, we find ourselves in such beautiful moments together celebrating love. We are all, in a sense, just travelling home! I like that catchy celebratory song by Norman Greenbaum, *Spirit in the Sky*. Jenni, Joy, Jacqui, and I, sing it with ukuleles. Also, we know that the biggest gift is the present, and loving each other makes connections sparkle.

Henry Drummond wrote, ***"You will find as you look back upon your life that the moments when you have truly lived are the moments when you have done things in the spirit of love."***

😇 This of course includes first loving ourselves despite all our human imperfections! None of us are perfect but being confident and focusing on being our best in all we do gives us peace and knowledge that we couldn't have done any better and we can celebrate that!

Longevity runs in both our families. I attribute this, not only to great genes, but to lifestyle, especially avoiding stress, tension, and worry. As a child, I prayed fervently that my grandparents would never die. I loved them so much. Our family was privileged to have my paternal grandmother, Lila Thomson, until 106 years of age. Nothing is more certain than death and taxes, so my world of wishes was not realistic! I do count her wonderful long life as a prayer come true and believe in eternal life.

When my paternal grandfather passed away, I was a young student nurse, and the training hospital wouldn't allow me time off for his funeral, as my allocated days off were gone. This was a pivotal point for me, learning firsthand about compassion. I wished I'd been bold enough to take sick leave. I also then told myself I wouldn't sing again because singing reminded me of the great joy it was to sit on his knee while milking cows, as he sang, *Santa Lucia, Goodbye Dolly Gray, Kiss Me Goodnight Sergeant-Major,* and *If You Were the Only Girl in the World*, which sometimes brought tears to his eyes. I wanted to wallow in misery at his passing. Gratitude, acceptance, and maturity really helped me grow beyond these constrained thoughts.

✝ Errol for years has said, "If I'd known I was going to live this long, I'd have looked after myself a lot better!" It's never too late to live boldly and have an audacious goal. It makes all the difference in how we navigate the twists and turns that life inevitably takes.

Forming new habits takes focus, persistence, and action. A lesson even in this reflection is to not waste energy thinking about what we haven't done and the goals we haven't achieved, but to send our thoughts to the outcomes we really want and powerfully act to make them happen.

Even in preparation for this book, Errol was triggered recalling distressing traumatic memories post brain surgery, when irritability, less tolerance, and notably, his newly trimmed already 'short wick' compounded in mania.

Sometimes, the brain does not like to revisit an unresolved disturbing past. It was gold for me to recognise after reminiscing, that acceptance is part of the journey of awakening. Rewiring thought patterns may be a key to dissolving distress from the past so that we see every day as a new opportunity for a fresh start. Experience and knowledge sure do shape us. Doing the Landmark Forum was transformative for me personally in this area, even though I already had made peace with the past, I cleared it for an infinitely incredible future of all possibilities.

The expectation is that our collective dreams will come true. When we put it into action, everything accelerates. Enthusiasm in action is the mother of success. It's easy to put our own spin on twisted threads and associations of memory, changing the meaning because of something we've carried deep and made true in our minds and then it's sealed again in spoken and written words. These days, I don't wish to open a Pandora's Box nor touch any old wounds unless hotwired with love and healing balm. It is what it is. Acknowledging what persistently returns and not reacting has healing power. Poking the bear in confrontation and getting that expected aggressive reaction is not worth it.

"Reducing all stress, toxicity and inflammation, getting good sleep, a little sunshine, good dentition, maintaining heart rate variability, insulins and a healthy mildly ketotic state via diet and exercise, optimises cognition for best brain health." Dr.Daniel G. Amen.

"Energy flows where attention goes." Tony Robbins

"Mastering love is key." Nurse Claire Voyant.

Empowerment from feeling unconditional love above the negativities has a definite and immediate positive impact on stress levels. Hey, you! Take a breath! Learn to let it go! Living abundantly begins with appreciation. I'm so grateful for all those near and dear to me. You matter so much. One of my mother's pearls is, "Now is the best time... Go and do it! Do it once and do it properly... not half pie!" I used to picture half a pie. In America I think they say, half-baked, others might say half-cocked. In Māori, Pai means good. The take-home was always to do it properly or not at all!

Half my life has been watching friends come and go over the horizon. Reciting the ancient Nicene Creed from my confirmation as a Christian, nursing those dying, and witnessing the miracle of birth and creation, lightens and affirms my belief in the spirit world and afterlife.

😇 Bishop Brent (1862 to 1926) wrote:

What is dying? *I am standing on the seashore. A ship sails in the morning breeze and starts for the ocean. She is an* *object of beauty and I stand watching her until at last she fades on the horizon and someone at my side says, "She is gone." Gone! Where? Gone from my sight, that is all. She is just as large in the masts, hull, and spas as she was when I saw her, and just as able to bear her load of living freight to its destination. The diminished size and total loss of sight is in me, not her, and just at the moment when someone at my side says, "She is gone" there are others who are watching her coming, and other voices take up a glad shout "There she comes!"–and that is dying.*

😇 I was also honoured to meet both of Siena's grandmothers, rest their souls. This special top-end family met ours at our annual Christmas get-together at Brunswick Heads, New South Wales. It's a true pleasure being in Siena's life as her special Saltwater-Sister, godmother come midwife and courtesy aunty, of course. I've watched stage and outdoor performances and dance competitions, listened in awe as she recited the entire periodic table to the tune of the *Can-Can*, and heard her speak on radio interviews and in podcasts. I'm in awe, not only of what she has achieved in her short life so far but of her potential, as she also understands that anything is possible and that she can do it as a modern and traditional Yolgnu woman!

We were delighted to be present for her 18th birthday celebrations at the Walkabout Hotel in Nhulunbuy on the Gove Peninsula, with a stylish black and white theme. I count it a privilege to have known Siena from the moment of birth and her first breath and I'm sure I was meant to be exactly where I was in the world on that auspicious day. I'm truly inspired to write this book because Siena, at age 14, and other friends and family, have inspired me by writing their own books and I have stories to share. Some shares will resonate with you mildly and some might just knock your socks off!

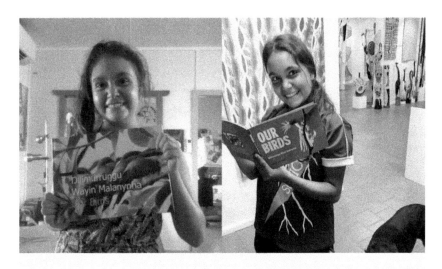

Siena Stubbs with an early version of Our Birds (left) and, two years later. *(Supplied: Will Stubbs)*

Miss Siena Mayutu Wurmarri Stubbs of the Gumatj clan of the Yirritja moiety.

The world really has become much smaller with advancing technology and cyberspace keeping us connected. I celebrate this sentimental journey home, knowing every choice has consequences. Options chosen may take time, energy, finances, discipline, courage, and lots more, yet ultimately, we are responsible for managing our own situations, making the best decisions we can contemporaneously, and involving ourselves in life, above watching it go by.

No man is an island. I believe living by the Volume of the Sacred Law and feeling gratitude as we benefit others through love makes the magic of success ours. Oh, sure we all have excuses or reasons and sometimes they're valid. Naivety, inexperience, age, coercion, time, weather, health, finances, priorities, and being in the right place at that time, can sometimes boost us when open to possibilities, as can letting go of persistent negatives that just pull us down. Ah, freedom and serenity! Others may only hold our hands for part of the journey. Most of our adventure routes have been instigated by Errol and I've followed, then taken him to roads less travelled, whilst being supportive.

♥ This book is an opportunity to share and shine love, give and get whatever guidance I can, and step up to the plate in whatever way helps others. Most of us are reared to tune in and act upon what love would do. I now filter things through the lens of the T.H.I.N.K. principle. Before speaking, ask if it is TRUE? HELPFUL? INSPIRATIONAL? NECESSARY? Is it KIND? Rule number one is to do no harm.

My own winning formula is a sentence of ten two-lettered words.

IF IT IS TO BE, IT IS UP TO ME.

😇 I will do my best to deliver this baby knowing nature has its own way and that others do already expect great things. There's a big responsibility that I'll hold myself accountable for, and some things that will be out of my hands, yet attainable through knowledge, understanding and acceptance of the unseen. Ah yes, God and his angels work in mysterious ways!

I'm grateful for courage and focused learning with trust and patience that my love, joy, hope, body, and mind's needs are already met. An awesome attitude is everything.

Being robbed of hope by a doctor is so life-threatening, yet holding hope can be a true lifesaver. "While there is breath, there is hope" (Dum Spiro Spero). We all die. We also usually want our chosen medics to prolong life. Errol's mother's journey, rest her soul, gave testimony to this, as she fulfilled her desire to live and be well at home for many months after discharge from palliative care, despite their plan. She knew she could, so she did! Take assertive action! Staying sharp is a valuable life skill that we can also influence.

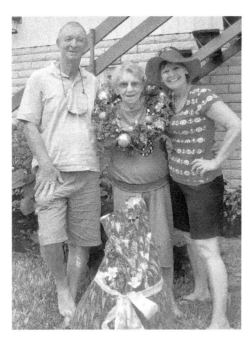

This true gift of love, cow dung hand-collected by my mother, sister, and me, directly from the footings of the old farm homestead near Bungawalbin Creek during our Parish family Christmas camp-out, delighted my mother in law, Nan, whose prize roses also benefitted.

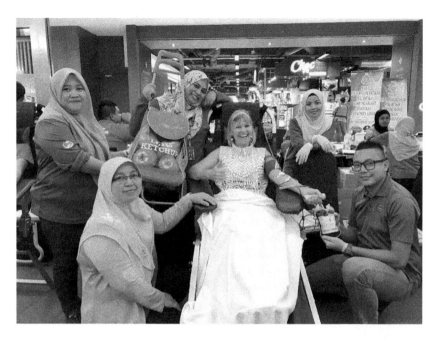

*Giving another gift that keeps on giving: B positive lifeblood
in Imago Shopping Centre Kota Kinabalu Borneo.*

My parents gave this gift of life 3 monthly in NZ until they were
deemed too old by law. ♥ The cycle of life will continue just as
it has for eons. Our understanding of it may change in a flash.
Birth – death; it's that dash of time and action between these life
events that also matters and is our measure of a life well-lived.
My life so far has been incredible, having now spent more time
living in Australia than in my homeland, New Zealand. I was
a tax-paying Australian citizen living aboard our boat for nearly
three decades. I also have a deep affinity for my motherland.
My heart is here with Errol, though, so I'm at home. Across the
Tasman Sea is a short flight.

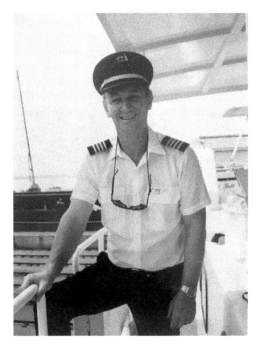

Captain Errol has flown his own aircraft to N.Z., refueling at Lord Howe and Norfolk Islands.

✚ Being a midwife with end-of-life palliative and hospice experience, I feel, has been sacred, helping keep me grounded and balanced. It's a privilege to be with another at birth and witness the miracle of life's first breath, and equally sacred being present at the final breath of death. None of us get out of this life alive! In between, I've loved Accident and Emergency Nursing. Resuscitation especially taught me, that life is a fine line and to avoid it flattening.

I really like the song *Perhaps Love* by John Denver. Maybe it'll be a funeral song, like Roger Whitacker's *The Last Farewell* and Graham Rodger's *Heart of the Kimberley*.

☺ Throughout my life, I have bargained and made promises to God, myself and others. "Oh God, help me pass this exam and I will follow your first command...", "Oh God don't let Mr. Woodley know I haven't practiced piano this week and I will do more...", "Oh Lord give me strength to be a better person!", and "Oh God help me make a difference!"

When gratefulness and confidence are part of these bargains and cries, there's a belief that hardship and good times will pass. Amen, and it's already done! With confidence, I have done my best for years, mostly with adequate preparation to maintain momentum and wing my way to success by being open to love and opportunities as they came my way. The common thread has been having a consistently brave enough attitude to put in the action of doing what must be done to get to the line in a kindly manner. Often, this has been under pressure from time constraints of leaving things to the last minute. Yes, sometimes winging it, once the groundwork is done, really is the key for me. There's a freedom that comes with being ready. How often, though, are we ever really ready for the major life changes that come our way? Self-doubt and comparison are well-known saboteurs. It's a trap as there are always greater and lesser than us. To those who judge, I want to say, "Learn the art of compassion, and go love yourself!"

😇 **Mother Theresa said,**
"If you judge people, you will have no time to love them."

🖤 I'm a can-do person. It's difficult to be anxious when grateful. Gratitude gives us freedom wings. It has taken me a long time not to worry about what others think. Now, I speak my truth more easily, knowing those who matter and love unconditionally, without judgement, will simply—with understanding—sift away any bad and hold the good, knowing that my heart is good and things have a way of working out for the best.

Being forgiving by nature and dropping all judgement frees us from the clutches of disease and resentment. Life really is too short to hold grudges. Getting relationships right sometimes just needs us to step out of our comfort zone and maybe make a bold request without fixing or changing while being honest and open. It may take some courage. Fully expressing our love without doubting is so powerful and so is restoring integrity when it's lost. Cleaning up is cathartic, ACTION IS POWER! Whatever brings peace of mind also brings happiness as a by-product. DOSE with those free feel-good hormones, dopamine, oxytocin, serotonin, and endorphins.

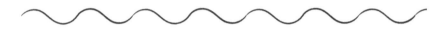

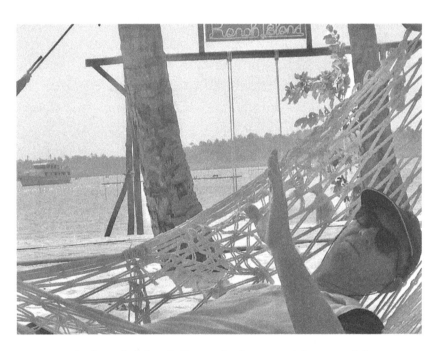

At Ranoh Island, Riau, Indonesia: After crayfish lunch: Rest a while, after dinner walk a mile.

CHAPTER 6

CLAIRE DE LUNE

 Claire means **light and bright.**

My happy childhood holds me in good stead. All parents want their kids to play nicely in life, even as adults. I love all my family unconditionally. Life's greatest blessing really is the love of family. This 'family' doesn't have to be biological. One of the biggest misconceptions I've heard is that blood makes you family. Blood makes you related…trust, loyalty, and unconditional love make you family. Generational blessings are a gold mine and can be defiled by misunderstandings and toxicity. Forgiveness keeps us in the fold. Life is lighter when we put our ego behind us choosing forgiveness. This stems from resentment, contempt and bleeding from 'deadly sins'… pride, lust, envy, anger, slothfulness (ego) gluttony and greed (my acronym; PLEASE Give Good). The rule of three comes back to me threefold. I love all my family and my Scottish and Irish roots. I love to laugh, believe good things are coming and pray for peace and wisdom.

Born the middle child to Harold and Margaret Thomson from Southbridge in the South Island of beautiful New Zealand, I will always love them and the great outdoors.

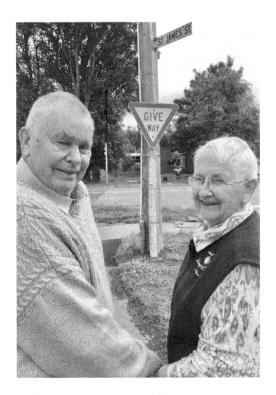

I honour, respect and love my parents.

I choose rose-coloured glasses, believing the world is full of beauty when hearts are full of love. My mother country has such natural beauty and opportunities for all. I love New Zealand's National Anthem lyrics of love, praise, unity, freedom, peace, protection, righteousness, truth, and glory to God. As children, by repetition, we learned the old version of the Lord's Prayer, prior to having any understanding of the words, or meaning:

Our Father who art in Heaven, hallowed be thy name, thy kingdom come, thy will be done, on earth as it is in Heaven. Give us this day our daily bread and forgive us our trespasses, as we forgive those who trespass against us. Lead us not into temptation but deliver us from evil. For thine is the kingdom, the power and the glory, forever and ever. Amen.

Old English is engrained in my brain. The understanding, the 10 commandments and so much more would come later.

At age seven, I became a Brownie Guide, standing before leaders and peers promising the law: "To think of others before myself and do a good turn every day." The motto, "Lend a Hand" taught me early to serve. At nine, I felt lucky to become a Girl Guide repeating, "I promise on my honour, to do my best, to do my duty to God, to serve the Queen and my country, to help other people and keep the Guide Law." The 10 laws briefly were to be trusted, loyal, useful, friendly, courteous, kind, obedient, cheerful, thrifty and pure of heart and mind. The Guide motto: "Be prepared" has also been a great motto to live by.

Good foundations were set by being true to these virtues, firstly within the family unit and in the wider world. To have the fruits of the spirit, I've learned the best way is to stay connected to the vine and learn from teachers, ascended masters, and enlightened beings of love and light with high vibration; Jesus, who said, "I am the way, the truth and the life," as well as Buddha, St Francis, Muhammad, Mother Mary, Moses, Vishnu and so on.

Ranger guides followed until general and obstetric nursing training took my time in Timaru. The Queen's Guide award bestowed on Her Majesty, Queen Elizabeth II's behalf by New Zealand's then Governor General, Sir Keith Holyoake, honoured me in preparation with endless opportunities. As a royalist, I now cry out, "Long Live the King!" I was loyal first to his mother, rest her soul. Her auspicious funeral date 19/09/22 heralded moving into our new home. My early experiences have certainly helped to shape my life believing I can do anything, and that the world is my oyster.

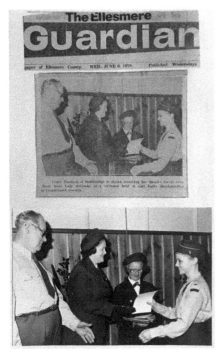

☺ We cannot control another's will and our promises may not always be fulfilled when reliant on another. Changing the goalposts and judgement in a different paradigm can help maintain our own integrity as "It's not a perfect world." Errol has reiterated this perspective of the world for years. Recognising the impact and doing our utmost to avoid similar disappointing repeats gives life itself the opportunity to send us some undreamed possibilities. For an idealist, disappointment can be devastating, oh but here lies the gift and the lesson. We keep learning that there's so much more to learn to really become transformed, to give this gift to others and live life skipping fantastically and tripping the light fandango into bliss.

🦋 Aspiring to be and act as a perfect being does sound moralistic. I believe my growth is part of the Master Planner of the Universe, Great Architect, Healer, Potter, God's Will, or Yoda-Yoda-Yoda! Yoda means wise, old and hero. I also thank God for protection, transformation, restoration, grace and for being so forgiving!

Ever conscientious (a real goodie-goodie!) at Southbridge District High School, when all five in my French class gave up, I continued via correspondence, learning the power of staying ahead with homework. Our first exchange student was the beautiful Tahitian Kiki. We laughed and learned a lot with her. Her father's cousin, Mrs. Dorothy Richards, a kindly woman, invited us home to a traditional Tahitian feast in Christchurch. Her conversation stayed with me for 48 years. I was 14, impressionable, with no idea what I would become. When she asked me, I answered, "Maybe I'll become a nurse or a teacher, I'm not sure yet." Immediately, her eyes lit up. She smiled, leaned in, saying, "Well, if you do become a nurse, you might go to Darwin and meet my daughter, Adrienne. She's a nurse at the Royal Darwin Hospital. That's in the Northern Territory, right up the top of Australia."

I had no idea of Darwin, and even Australia was so far away. The following year, the Languages Association of NZ sponsored me as an exchange student to visit idyllic French Polynesia. I went to Kiki Brotherson's home on the outlaying leeward island of Raiatea. It was a life-changing experience living with these beautiful friendly Polynesians and my heart thanks all the international yachties who also opened theirs, inspiring me with world travel and endless possibilities for living an extraordinary life on the path less travelled.

One family, the Kohuts from Ventura California, had their yacht, 37-foot "Getel" moored at Uturoa Yacht Club. Their daughters, 10 and 8, and 16-year-old nephew, Eric Rigney, were enrolled at the local school. Eric and I were mostly in different classes but occasionally lunched together to speak English, then walked home after school, again laughing, and joking in English. It was so good for my brain to turn off. He was funny. His American accent was strong and he took the mickey out of my Kiwi twang. Written French was one thing, but the spoken word seemed so fast and foreign. I kept in touch with Eric about every two to five years via postcards, then we sent messages in a bottle to and fro.

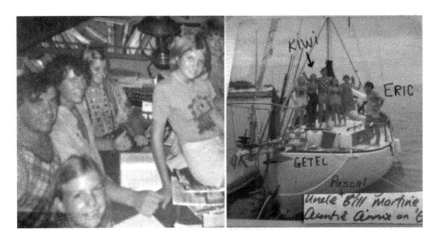

SY Getel's American family inspired my cruising life. Thank you

The nostalgia of friendship that spans four decades—from walking home together speaking English after school as teens in Uturoa Raiatea, me as a Kiwi exchange student and Eric as a deckhand, realising how our lives are influenced by others living theirs to the full, and how dreams to go cruising can and do (SY Kandu, Idlewise/MY Restless M) come true in our own corners of the world and then together in the really big pond. It's a small world after all, and our reunion at Sail

Malaysia's rally, after not seeing each other in over 25 years, is a big heart story that I love to share! Thank you Rigney family. Thank you Raiatea Magic and Great Architect of the Universe (GAOTU) for teaching us to wish upon a star, put in action and make dreams come true.

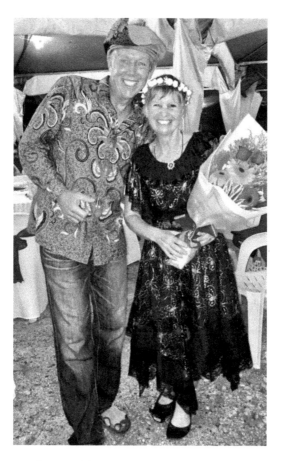

Wearing the sparkly green and gold butterfly lace dress that Eric and Leslie returned to Mexico to purchase for me, some 31 years ago, as the little shop had closed early the day I went, preventing my anticipated purchase. It arrived in Canada with their Eiffel Tower proposal movie, surprising me hugely. I cried with joy at their kindness.

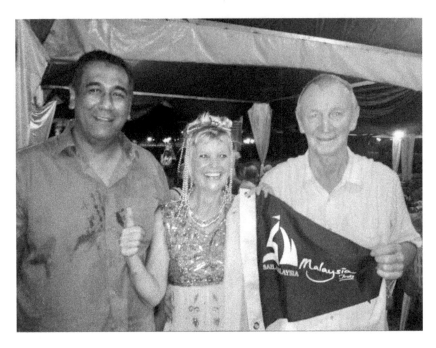

*With our highly esteemed Sail Malaysia organiser Sazli
at another Pankor Island Marina rally dinner.*

As a teenager in a foreign land, I was busy, yet wrote some 'I miss you' letters to my boyfriend in Rakaia, New Zealand, describing life in French Polynesia. I wrote articles for our local rag, *The Ellesmere Guardian,* and I took my time abroad seriously to be the best ambassador for New Zealand possible. The learning curve was overwhelming. I went out surfing near the reef and got a shark fright so I stayed aboard the runabout becoming seasick. Staying at a beautiful motu (islet), I experienced melting into cane peacock chairs. I love stretches of tropical cumulous clouds just above the horizon, azure crystal-clear water, balmy breezes and sunsets.

I bonded well with Pappa Rasmus who made great ice cream and delicious pineapple pie. Fondly I remember sailing across to

Tahaa Island with him from Raiatea. They share one coral reef. Sunburn got me and the thrill of sailing far from shore. I had no fear and the Hobie-cat sail was divine. My cousin Rebecca, who was schooling in Papeete, visited us. She struggled with the language. A very nasty, painful, slow-healing tropical ulcer was deep on her shin, stopping her from swimming.

We flew as a family to Bora Bora and Huahine to visit more families. There was always a lot of laughter, food and fantastic music with drums, great guitars, amazing ukuleles and dancing. My blonde hair was a novelty for young men. I soon learned to do the Tahitian waltz. Memorable too was dancing with my younger sister, Tiare, every night just before TV news when the Tahitian drums would fast beat the traditional Tamure. We would swing into Tahitian dancing, hips gyrating super-fast, shoulders not moving, arms out wide and feet flat on the floor. Practice makes perfect.

A fan of summer in NZ, I loved blackberrying, cycling, camping, tramping, canoeing, tennis, water skiing and netball. You name it, I would be in like Flynn! (that's Errol Flynn). Picking raspberries for my Uncle Ken and Auntie Alice with other cousins during summer holidays made good pocket money. It seemed like a competition; whoever could pick the fastest, best quality was rewarded with the best pay packet, and we could eat as many as desired. I couldn't overindulge. Bliss!

My brother Bruce cut our long driveway hedge fortnightly for 50 cents. I did it when he played team sports. My weekly pocket money was 10 cents, his was 15 cents. Our tasks differed. I learned early that sometimes it pays to do what we don't really want early (like peeling potatoes before school while he prepared firewood). I babysat two days per week after school, preparing another family's dinner for 20 cents. Returning bottles gave good refunds, although we rarely found them as our small town was tidy. Hedge trimming was ideal for suntanning, daydreaming and blisters from the wooden handles. There was less growth in winter and more daydreaming of the Pacific Islands! I saw my future self in halter-neck white bathers on the bow of a big white boat! I dreamed of the escape, created it and realised it fully! I learned the proverb: look after the pennies and the pounds look after themselves and be careful what you wish for!

🙂 There was no special treatment for girls at Southbridge District High School either, and the threat of being caned by respected science teacher Mr Stewart Gavin was taken so seriously that I stopped crocheting under his science lab desk immediately as warned! I was proud of the double bedspread I made mostly in his class. Humiliation and fear worked for me.

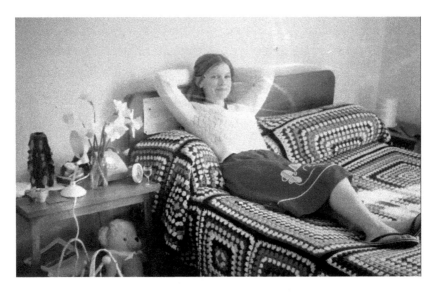

Crafty crochet almost had me caned in class!

Other teachers have also made massive impacts on my personality and education. I praise the wonderful Woodleys and aspire to have happy wrinkles like Mrs. Woodley's love lines. She had a lovely sparkle in her blue eyes which may have reflected from her mesmerising crystal beads. I now call them love crystals and Myrtle beads. Her name symbolised love, affection and beauty. She was also kind and approachable. Kids pick up on these qualities. I was, however, nervous I'd be found out for not practicing piano by her husband, who was later also diagnosed with Parkinson's Disease. He told my parents they were wasting their money if I didn't do the required practice! Music tuition was a luxury not afforded to all.

My mother's clever psychology to encourage piano practice was delegating the evening washing up to my siblings, Bruce, and Anthea, simultaneously instructing by pointing for me to go and practice. Initially, I wasn't happy, but I soon learned this meant escaping the mundane, and I'm ever so grateful to my mum for her perseverance. Making music is a big part of my life. The gift keeps on giving. Years later, I played for Mr Woodley in his nursing home and we both appreciated the learning and the listening.

The 'temper' of one relieving primary school teacher, through tears, taught me about patience and compassion, especially toward children. I still talk a lot though, ha-ha! It wasn't healthy coming home unhappy from feeling 'picked on'. My brother was bullied at school. It was very memorable for us all. Succinctly and gently confronting this same hair-pulling bully at our school's 100-year celebration was satisfying. I prefer confrontation avoidance, yet ensured he understood accountability to me and my brother for his meanness, despite us all being children.

My younger sister Anthea's dream came true with Toby, her first pony. She learned discipline, responsibility, bonding and she loves horses. Watching 12-year-old Bruce dragged by one stirrup around the back paddock gave me healthy respect. I've fallen and gotten back up, learning that water is more forgiving than sky or land.

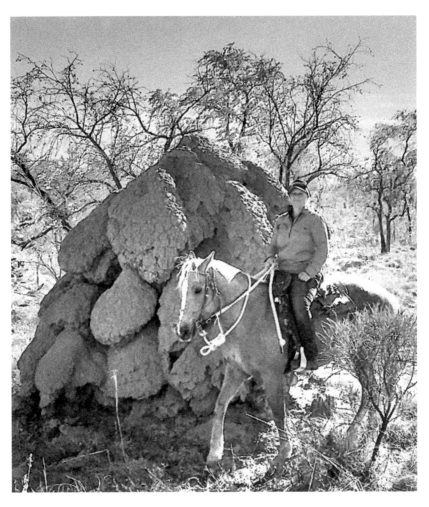

Sister Anthea on "The Blonde" along the Gibb River Road, Western Australia.

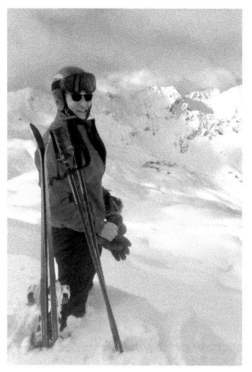

Brother Bruce in his element at Rainbow Skifield, New Zealand

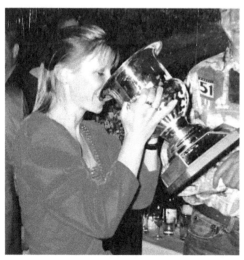

I celebrate life!

Our small farming community only had a couple of Māori families, and the Ngai Tahu Marae (meeting house) at Taumutu was about 15 km from Southbridge. Music, art, and Māori culture were gifted to us by Mrs. Brown from Taumutu. She requested I play piano at morning assembly several times. Obliging, terribly nervous and quivering in front of about 100 pupils and teachers, I'd reluctantly become a people pleaser.

Dutchman Mr. Meissen taught French and history. We got on well. Notably, he smoked a pipe along the corridors for years. Mr. Banks was always proper in his manner and delivery of geography and social studies, except when a drone missile (blackboard duster) was directed at bad boys. Teachers mentored us and we gratefully remember their gems, offered by their own example of respect and character. Some mathematics teachers could easily be distracted by requests for their wartime stories on land and sea.

Awaiting nursing training, childcare and local horticulture rewarded me. Working in very large glass houses, mainly cross-pollinating, then outside planting cabbages and picking strawberries, potatoes and tomatoes was great exercise but backbreaking.

✝ I proudly became a New Zealand Registered General and Obstetric Nurse, but not before learning the huge lesson of overcoming failure. A surprising number in our class failed first state exams. My lovely godparents sent a beautiful bouquet, followed by apologies for their perceived salt-in-the-wound action. We were all surprised. I consolidated training, specialising in endocrinology in cold old Dunedin. I cycled lots, despite the ice, wearing an array of wild headgear and gloves and was saved by the smell from Cadbury's chocolate factory.

I saw an advertisement for dog, cat and house-minding. Soon my nursing girlfriend Rachael and I moved into a large Tudor-style 'Belmont House', on Belmont Lane, above Anderson's Bay, Dunedin. In lieu of rent, we also de-cobwebbed and dusted the chandeliers and the 20-seater dining table, vacuumed, and ensured the tassels were straight on all the Persian mats. The owner often travelled overseas, so we had the entire run of English sheepdog Bazil and the cold house. We chose our own bedrooms and lounge room upstairs and hosted great dinner parties with roaring fires!

My room had a glorious, big, wide, bay window overlooking Dunedin harbour. I delighted in the twinkling lights on the

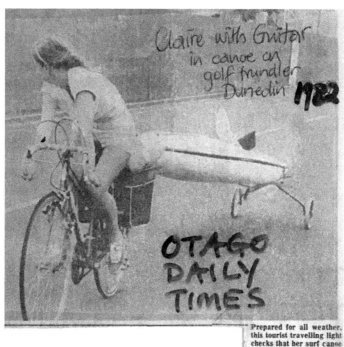

Claire with Guitar in canoe an golf trundler Dunedin 1982

OTAGO DAILY TIMES

Prepared for all weather, this tourist travelling light checks that her surf canoe is still following as she cycles along Victoria Road yesterday.

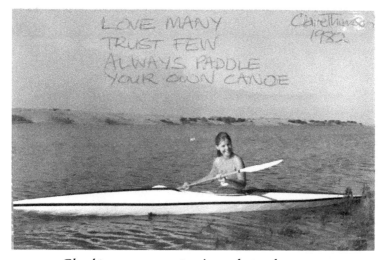

LOVE MANY
TRUST FEW
ALWAYS PADDLE
YOUR OWN CANOE

Claire...
1982

Checking on my guitar's angle in the canoe.

opposing hills reflected in the water at night-time as I lay on my belly, level with the window. When off-duty, I often towed my canoe on a modified golf trundler behind my pushbike. Yes, a head-turning functional conversion. Professional tasting evenings when our wines and spirits sales manager returned were fun as was visiting the underground cellar. Maybe I developed delusions of grandeur back then, purchasing a ¾ length grand piano for our upstairs lounge room! It came from a nunnery and was only played by virgins, or so my dad said! Life is like a piano, what you get out of it depends on how you play it! After nursing consolidation and first love abandonment, I planned my return to beautiful Tahiti.

Thankfully, my parents babysat my piano for decades, then various NZ friends. A cloth template helped visualise pending positioning aboard Restless M before the shipment arrived in Port Brisbane, Australia. The legs and stool were temporarily lost in transit, so it arrived 'legless', upsetting me greatly. Eureka! Exhale! The crate was forklifted aboard on its side onto the back deck, castors removed, then the piano was hand-carried through aft doors onto our new saloon's carpet by 8 Maritimo shipyard men.

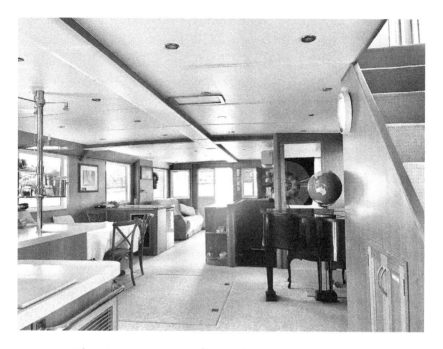

The piano was initially in the aft saloon near the cockpit, and later was moved forward nearer the dining area. I loved playing whilst cruising.

⚓ Sea trials were prior to bolting piano legs down with stainless steel adjustable stays. Four of us headed out around Cape Moreton, re-entering the Broadwater via Gold Coast Seaway. Nasty conditions with swell caused yaw, roll and three of us to hold that piano. Despite its deadweight, it rocked and tipped. I prayed for the strength of those eight men and vanished visions of *The Piano* crashing below through to the double cabin, the hull, and further to the bottom of the sea like in the movie. Entry into the Broadwater was rough. Three mortals and strong nun spirits steadied my 'baby'. Lesson: battening down early is always prudent.

It was ironic having my piano aboard a boat, after years of over-protection. It practically sang out, "Just play me!" Red-felt fabric covering strings helped keep out salt air. Surprisingly, it's tune held very well. The piano now resides in our new home.

✛ Nursing took me to many work places and I was prepared to extend myself. I had an amazing post-graduate variety in these specialist units, areas and wards—spinal, physical disability, psychiatric—specialising in electro-convulsive therapy, burns, same-day procedures, hyperbaric medicine, intensive care, coronary care, acute general medical assessment, neonatal intensive care, rapid assessment, post-operative recovery, lots of accident and emergency departments, medical wards, endocrinology, infectious-Avian flu and Tuberculosis, respiratory, rehabilitation, obstetrics and gynaecology, midwifery, children's general and children's infectious, palliative care, and surgical wards, plus aged care homes, antenatal education, and hospice.

Multiple nursing agencies taught prioritorising and adaptation. Relieving as RNRM, and living in the matron's quarters above Kaikoura Hospital New Zealand was a huge responsibility in the maternity, and aged care units of two co-joined wings. Flying and grass strip arrival in a two-seater Agcat Biplane from Christchurch, kelp and scallop diving was also exciting there.

I was a locum occupational health and safety RN at the world's second-largest zinc-lead and silver deposit, at Macarthur River Mine near Borroloola, Northern Territory. It was challenging and again, I took responsibility seriously. The mine has now been converted from underground to open-cut.

I nursed in a cosmetic surgeon's clinic in Tahiti and escorted, with a resuscitation backpack, many patients on interstate flights for specialised surgeries in Australia. Orthopaedics was my least favoured area. I've seen many broken bones, including compound fractures.

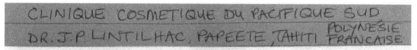

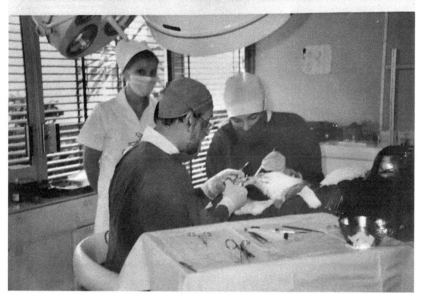

Observing a facelift by Dr J.P.Lintihac as scout. Volcanic mountainous views from our balcony overlooking a nightclub kept me appreciatively alert.

I probably witnessed more caesareans than any student midwife, as I love this life miracle, and took witness opportunities while with the anaesthetist. A nursing girlfriend once performed an emergency caesarean on a dying sheep, saving the lamb. Yes, Wendy! Years later, she gave healing touch (H.T.) complementary therapy, to my mother. Bless her and her hands. Confidence teaches us we can turn our hands with purpose to whatever the mind directs.

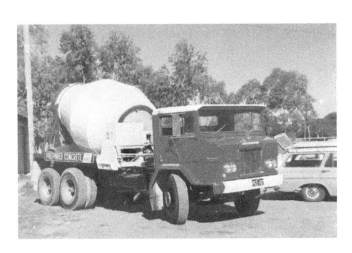

Caption: Errol's success was set in concrete, as he turned his mind and hands to making engines purr.

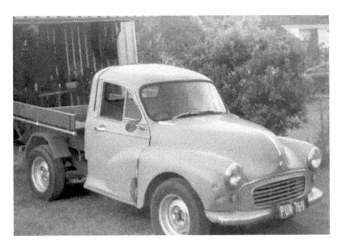

This ute was one in a collection of Errol's 14 Morris Minors.

CHAPTER 7

LIFE BEFORE ERROL AND B.C. (BEFORE CLAIRE)

✝ Before Claire (B.C.), Errol was a traveller and adventurer. He was back in Darwin after months in the Kimberley with fly-in and fly-out friends when we first met at the Sailing Club. He prepared Idlewise, as a radio relay vessel for his first International Darwin to Ambon Yacht Race. Before Errol, I also had an interesting adventurous life, and together, we continue an amazing life living outside the box.

Ten years before meeting Errol, I'd set off brokenhearted at 23 on my first big overseas experience visiting international friends. I returned to French Polynesia, immersed myself in the culture and when confident enough to fluently speak on the telephone, I drove to a night-nurse position in Dr. Jean Paul Lintilhac's cosmetic surgery clinic in Papeete. Life was expensive in Tahiti. Being a young bilingual registered nurse sealed the job. Clients wondered if I'd also been under the knife. The central Papeete operating theatre boasted spectacular views of peaky volcanic mountains and palm trees through glass sliding doors.

My achy-breaky heart mended. I was a young, naïve, idealist, placing extra significance on the biblical so-called 'man of my youth'. This decade-older doctor had pursued me relentlessly, from my steady boyfriend, in my second year of nursing. I devoted and pledged myself to this career-frustrated, complex, antisocial, double-minded Australian for 10 years believing I was the one for him. He was an aggressive hunter, enjoying the thrill of the chase, accruing many weapons, and notches with attitude. I was a blinded trophy. Dreams can fail mid-flight, and his rejection, for another, rocked my dreams.

Time was ripe for new friendship, meeting a tall, dark and handsome Englishman mid-flight, still laden with gifted, heavy shell necklaces, farewelling Tahiti for Apia, Western Samoa. This was the stopover for Tonga, where I'd meet with parents and Godparents volunteering service abroad. Two days sightseeing with Englishman, Paul, was easy. I was impressed he'd previously sailed to Samoa from beautiful Aitutaki in the Cook Islands, and he knew his way around, so I booked into the same safe, cheap, clean guest house and enjoyed his easy-going company, pleasant nature, kind eyes and smile. Especially memorable were the markets and visiting Robert Louis Stevenson's grave.

As he was bound for New Zealand, I shared my small travel brag book showcasing NZ. He quizzed me on the guy seen in many photos and bet a bottle of champagne I would marry this chap someday. I immediately, bet him a crate of champagne, I would not! Our flights to Tonga were one day apart, so we met at Nuku'alofa's post office. My parents had a spare room, so my new friend was welcomed into the fale (house).

An opportunity came for overnight travel by supply ship north to paradise, Ha'apai islands. Arriving by outrigger at the very small, untouched Foa Islet, I circumnavigated barefoot while dinner was cooked underground (in umu) then said, "How idyllic. What a shame we're not in love!" Then my lens became rosy. No tango for two in Tonga! Our issued tickets to NZ were on different dates, so we met again in Auckland before my return home to the South Island for work. He stayed north for work. My time was long whilst waiting for Paul the Pom but brief in the grand scheme of things.

Again I was chased by the persistent Aussie hunter and persuaded to rejoin him, as he apparently knew what was best for me. He also knew I'd met a strong suitor. I believe Paul's hopeful heart was very bruised (his parents rang me from England checking on my decision). My hand was forced to write the difficult 'Dear John' letter as directed and censored by the Aussie. I didn't recognise the control he had over me already.

Many of my nursing class were already married and I'd felt jilted, after four years of devotion, I was now swept off my feet and easily persuaded, without a proper proposal, to visit a Sydney jeweller, and wear his choice of sparkler, soon losing the bet for a crate of champagne. Third time lucky up the aisle he went. He accepted a part-time anaesthetic position at the Derby Regional Hospital and part-time with the Royal Flying Doctor Service (RFDS) in Western Australia (WA). So, I farewelled my family and friends for this adventure. My teenage fairytale dreams had come true, and the whirlwind bride ride began.

✝ The great Aussie outdoors was harsh after lush New Zealand and tropical paradise islands. I was unable to nurse as I was married to a hospital employee, said Matron, despite having WA nursing registration, being on-site, and rearing to work. Glossy interstate advertisements offered bonuses for nurses to go to Derby, WA. It was both incredulous and devastating. "Nothing personal," said Matron. Ha! It felt personal! 'Marital discrimination' was clearly the case agreed Dawn, the Commissioner for Anti-discrimination and Equal Opportunities in Perth, WA.

I wasn't very assertive back then, but my anaesthetist spouse was. Matron didn't like his 'bad gas' and manners. It was mutual. Over 2000 jobs were advertised with few applicants, so there were opportunities galore. I embraced Derby, living life fully. Meanwhile, only two RFDS clinics and three theatre lists per week materialised, and he loathed being sent to work in casualty.

My character developed. I was involved in the community. I babysat, joined the Uniting Church, and started my own Girl Guide company after seeing a stack of uniforms. I made advertising posters, found a venue, gathered the troop, and had fun. I grew veggies, played tennis, badminton, a couple of pianos, mud rugby, cycled everywhere, bird-watched, sketched, painted, kept house, baked and enjoyed learning to fly, plus went off camping every weekend.

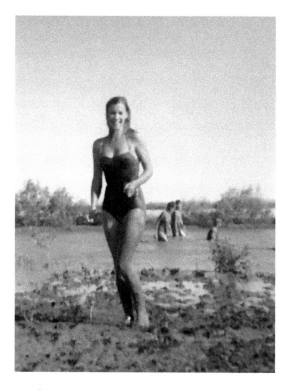

*Mud Rugby in Derby was great exercise and
fun. Ear plugs would have been prudent.*

A free, air-conditioned, furnished house, car and fuel card were
supplied. Camping required travelling many miles up the badly
rutted, dusty Gibb River Road beyond Meda Station, the King
Leopold Ranges, Mt Barnett Station and past the Napier Ranges
to amazing places like Tunnel Creek, Windjana and Geikie
Gorges. Exploring this great red land was fabulous. Winding
up windows fast at the last minute and slipping onto the grassy
verge whenever a truck passed was a fun, dusty race.

While the usual manager of the nearby new King Sound Hotel's
coffeeshop was away prospecting for gemstones, I ran it, easily

WHO'S IN CHARGE, MY BRAIN OR ME? (OR MY WIFE...)

selling my black forest cake and scones. There were hundreds of jobs available, so I could be selective.

Derby is a coastal outpost town, situated right up the King Sound with a very long winding jetty. Ships no longer use the port as some had come to grief from massive 12- to 15-metre tidal drops and fast, challenging rips. Flying lessons became too expensive to justify. I was grounded. Still loving sunset silhouettes especially. I was free to be me.

One paddock away from our medico's compound was Elder's, the general and agricultural store. It was soon bought by Woolworths, so I became their checkout chick, adding to my resume's highlights. Ringers from the stations bought clothing, hats, belts, buckles, music tapes and slabs of drinks. Provisions included large quantities of Nicky-Nicky (chewing tobacco) Tally Ho papers for rolling cigarettes, Log Cabin Tobacco, star pickets, lots of flour, tea, sugar, jam, and gas. It was also great for nurse-me receiving everybody's, "Hello, how are YOU today?" greetings.

I learned a lot about Aborigines despite their personal distance. Their catchy, easily identifiable, often biblical names fascinated me. Staff had no special indigenous training. It was learned by experience. Aboriginals were often misjudged through a lack of cultural awareness and understanding. They didn't make eye contact; most didn't speak my language and I certainly didn't speak theirs. They were tough, wiry and generally didn't present at the hospital unless gravely ill. I also learned a lot about alcohol and violence. Revenge payback violence was very strong in this culture. I saw sepsis from speared thighs, skull fractures from nulla nullas (hard clubs) some amazing 'sorry scars' from self-mutilation during grieving, infected tribal initiation circumcisions and healed yet out-of-shape limbs. Police followed up on screams from women in trouble beyond our compound. Looking back, general shouting about town could've been from deafness, as many tribal Aborigines had untreated ear infections as kids.

Years later, I house-minded, by chance, in Darwin, NT for the kind woman who supported me in raising my case when I couldn't nurse in Derby, WA. Our actions paved the way to help others before moving to the Northern Territory. A satisfying small-world story!

Western Australia's amazingly rugged and remote coastal Kimberley territory would, in another chapter of my life, recapture my heart and become a passionate cruising ground for over 20 years with Captain Errol. First came some life lessons.

The timing was good to leave Derby to meet new colleagues at the Royal Darwin Hospital, having been persuaded to join the annual end-of-year entertainment called "The Hospital Review". Despite initial shyness on stage, I was soon in my element. This show was a series of skits taking the mickey out of the hospital, the health system, and us as health workers.

 I met many colleagues with joy thanks to the Review's great lessons in not taking ourselves too seriously. Doctors aren't Gods. Nurses, though, are angels. I loved full-time nursing, beginning in a surgical ward specialising in eye surgery, and learning a lot in the burns unit. Campfires and alcohol aren't a good mix, and wounds healed slowly. Cafeteria food was good and cheap so made things easy when working. I grew a fabulous garden in the staff village and was active and sporty.

During one shift changeover, I farewelled an excited nurse about to collect holiday photographs and asked her where? She responded, "Tahiti!"

Instantly, I commented, "Oh beautiful! I love French Polynesia! Did you get to any outlaying or Leeward islands?"

She was surprised that I even knew of Tahiti! I added I have family there.

"So do I!" she responded.

I told her my family lives on Raiatea Island, in Uturoa.

"That's where my family lives!" she exclaimed.

I noted her star-shaped, burgundy-bordered enamel New Zealand nurse's medallion. She asked what the surname of my family was. I replied, "Brotherson."

She gasped in excitement, "Who? Who?"

I replied, "Rasmus Brotherson."

"He's my uncle!" she said.

My brain joined the memory dots and I simply blew her away asking, "Is your mother Dorothy Richards from Christchurch?"

"YES! Mum will be flying over to Darwin in 10 days, so come to Nightcliff Road and see her one afternoon for tea!"

I did, and 10 years melted away.

I became a Brownie Leader at Malak, NT. Organising fun programmes and shaping girls with enthusiasm and confidence was especially rewarding. (Midwifery is, essentially, the empowerment and care of childbearing women, newborns, and families.) Together we learned the national anthem, sang and tape-recorded, "Happy Birthday Grannie from Darwin NT, Skippy and me," to the tune of *Waltzing Matilda*. I hired a kangaroo suit from Sydney's Abracadabra store and hopped over to New Zealand to celebrate Grannie's 90th birthday. The faux fur roo suit had independently moveable ears operated by hidden cords below chest level, an ample pouch for Minties, reddish claws on its paws, and a long tail to lift and swing. The realistically molded Kangaroo head sat on top of mine. Our cat went berserk on dress rehearsal at the moving ears! Despite self-consciousness, I lowered the roo's head at Grannie's party and surprised everyone. Sometimes, the fear of looking silly or of not being enough (or being too much!) is overcome by making others happy.

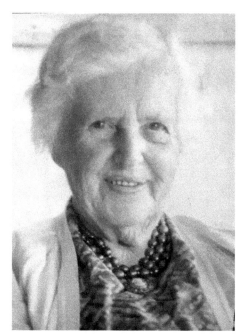
Grannie Lila Thomson so loved.

✝ Any weekends off were spent camping at Kakadu and life was busy in between. Working in Accident and Emergency (A&E) in Darwin was rewarding. Nurses did everything and back then, the territory's population was generally younger, impacting what people presented with. Life, health, and death were not taken for granted, despite the gun-ho, bulletproof vibe of youth.

Within the framework of a great team, I felt totally supported and confident, learning to take blood, insert IV lines, suture lacerations, remove fishhooks, resuscitate, and stabilise victims of car accidents, assaults, croc and snake bites, Irukandji jellyfish stings, bull and buffalo gorings, fractures, burns, rashes, sprains, pain, and drug use. We also redressed wounds, managed pregnant women and drunks, and supported children, the elderly, and people with mental health challenges, sporting injuries, and other troubles. There was plenty to learn and laugh about, including ourselves.

I considered working for the Aeromedical Service. Midwifery was a requirement, so we transferred to Alice Springs temporarily for his work and my training. The Darwin A&E and midwifery staff were great colleagues, keen to share, learn and teach. We remain close. Respectful relationships were built with the NT Police too. They brought in bakery goodies, and we made them midnight and beyond coffees. Friendships were forged with off-duty socialising at what was called weekly "Choir Practice" with a wind-down cricket game immediately after the Saturday night shift. Many police surprise-visited sergeant friend, Boots (RIP), for his 50th birthday party held at home, greatly intimidating the resident gun collector.

Accepting a radiographer's request to babysit, the address and home seemed familiar. It was the previous home of Kiwi Nurse Adrienne. This place later became my base in Darwin for years, and my relationship with the Nightcliff Road family remains strong. The four-year-old girl I'd babysat, decades later, came aboard, cruising up to Indonesia in 2016, then Malaysia, re-joining us in Thailand. Such warm fuzzies I feel for this family who were also there for me when the chips were down.

At 28, a student midwife, soon to start a family upon graduation, I was instead starting out again on my own. My then-husband, while I worked, took his new then 'soul mate' camping. I was so trusting and naïve. The concern my parents had about his previous marriages and behaviour affecting his future performance was justified. His 'philandering again', as his mother termed it, was a shattering shock. Promises, like bones, are not made to be broken. It happens and usually hurts. His hypocritic ego couldn't accept that I'd met another, after his rejection back when I was single, gaslighting me for years in our marriage. I had become subordinate. Now I recognise narcissism. I knew I was enough, yet still felt I'd allowed a marriage failure when it clearly takes two, sometimes three. Alone, I faced fear and was strong. Overcoming heartbreak takes time and courage. I cried, then stopped the luxury of self-pity partying knowing my faith was strong too and I would be OK.

Over time, my gratefulness increased for such a lucky escape as there were no children involved. Karma and weapons eventually ignited this gasman's consequences at Her Majesty's Service. Managing relationships is mostly learned by experience. Now all the help in the world is at our fingertips and we control the trigger action. What we tolerate, we perpetuate. I thank God now for his 'cyclical monogamy'. It gave me my life and freedom back albeit with some lessons. I became a registered midwife, did the family planning course, learned to sail, windsurf and dive, enjoying also the new skill of hyperbaric chamber nursing, whilst house-minding to better save for Plan B's sailing passage to Papua New Guinea (PNG) and world airfares. Half the money, twice the fun!

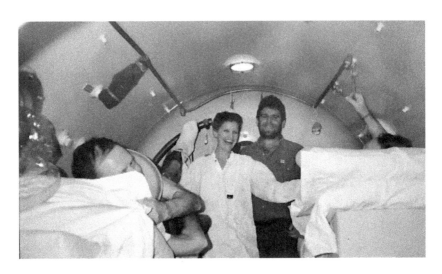

*Practicing Hyperbaric Medicine in Darwin
with Technician David King.*

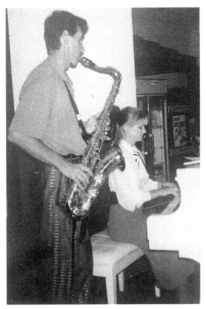

*Playing piano in public at
The Cool Spot- Fannie Bay
helped my nerves in time
for Mum's surprise 50 th*

124

After wound-licking hibernation, I was set up with a Northern Territory Parks and Wildlife Ranger on a blind date. My jealous ex arrived at our old hospital accommodation unit aggressively possessive, yet he lived with his mistress. Soon after, in the lecture auditorium, a medico tapped me on the shoulder, congratulating me on being pregnant. It wasn't me. My heart sank. Then I somehow allowed that estranged husband, just after he completed a pregnancy termination theatre list, to cry on my shoulder as his then 'soulmate'-mistress miscarried in Sydney when visiting her husband. How others treat us is their karma, how I respond is up to me.

He pursued her hard and his written in absence, Darwin Hospital resignation was accepted. He called himself a 'degenerate reprobate' and his wayward heart also broke his mother's good heart. She wrote to me when he was 'away', telling me his guns and woman had got him there. A lucky escape for me indeed.

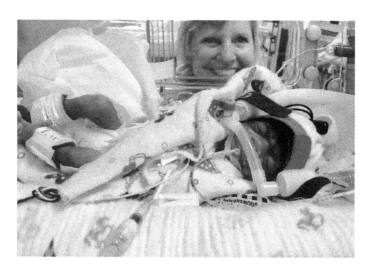

Neonatal Intensive Care nursing in Darwin was stressful in many personal ways and understandably I requested not to work there while my anaesthetist husband's new lover, a visiting paediatric registrar, was there.

Slowly, the world became a pearl. I loved the exciting ranger outdoors lifestyle on my days off. The first outing was croc catching up the east arm of Darwin Harbour with a well-known catcher, then helicopter-and bull-catcher mustering buffalo and wild horses, hydrofoil skimming over wetlands, 4WD patrolling for wild pigs and cats, monitoring duck shooters' licences, snakes, frogs and crocs, mainly around Fogg Dam Bird Sanctuary. Assisting in the annual data collection day at Janamba Crocodile Farm nearby meant bravely picking up crocs younger than two years, shorter than one metre, and rubber banding their jaws for the data analysts. Adrenaline ran high when one got loose. They have razor-sharp teeth. I loved this lifestyle and his family but chose not to stick with the ranger.

I bought around-the-world tickets, then met a dairy farmer when water skiing in New Zealand prior to delivering my sister Anthea's second-born son, Adam. Yes, it's very deep and meaningful to witness family birth. I flew to Europe via Tahiti. London was a great European hub, and I stayed at my cousin's in East Finchley, London where our grandfather had also lived. Ice creams and fantasising about the dairy farmer were travel treats. From Los Angeles again, I sent many tantalising personalised souvenirs so he couldn't forget me easily. After three weeks of sightseeing around Washington, D.C., I attended an International Hyperbaric Conference. Roberta Flack sang at the Washington Memorial, then a big, winged Pontiac took four backpackers and me up to New York for Independence Day celebrations.

We saw the Statue of Liberty, views from the World Trade Centre and fireworks from Brooklyn Bridge. Upon my NZ return, the heart-throb younger dairy farmer had strayed and was with a grand cougar instead of waiting for me. His dog had been run over in winter, and the vet nurse who looked after his dog looked after him too, more than I had! (wink-wink!) Lucky for me! Next! Swiss Rick from the NY Pontiac road trip arrived in NZ. He was drop-dead gorgeous through and through and I loved showing NZ off. As Whitney sang Dolly Parton's lyrics, I will always love you, the time came for him to travel on. Turning breakdowns into breakthroughs is a game-changer. I still feel the magic of synchronicity and serendipity, love, hope and joy and love learning. The hard way teaches resilience!

House-minding back in Christchurch helped me buy a character home with large gardens and fruit trees to keep me grounded. I

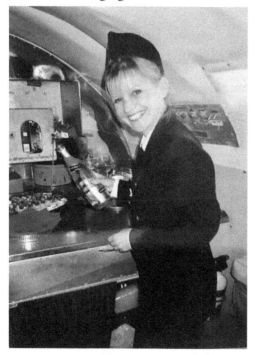

floated in the spa daily. Getting the bank loan was easy enough as I had eight and a half days of nursing work available per week on paper, plus DC3 flights, and two rooms direct-debit rented to family members.

Hostie me loved Champagne flights, dressing 1940's style, playing Boogie Woogie music and flying over beautiful N.Z.

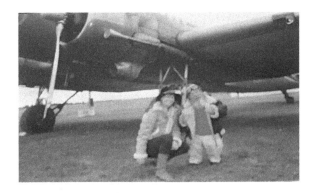

Hostessing with Pionair DC3 was one of the best jobs I ever had.
Santa Bob RIP from Mapua dressed as Biggles for his joy flight.

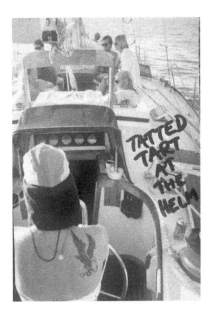

This temporary tatoo temporarily shocked my parents!

I took up gliding and ground-crewed in NZ during World Gliding Competitions at Omarama, for the Australian Champion, a 747 pilot. Although single, other interests elsewhere made him too complex! Instead of being blinded and burning more than the sun, I grew my own garden. Whilst weeding one day, I realised my youth could disappear right there or whilst making grape juice or jam! It was time to act. I escaped winter using those world frequent flyer points for another Darwin-Ambon Yacht race fix. I wasn't lost but was found by Errol in 1995.

CHAPTER 8

CAPTAIN MEETS HOT CAN-CAN KIWI

Errol and I met at the Darwin Sailing Club before an annual Darwin to Ambon Yacht Race. It was memorably Bastille Day, 1995 and my friend Debbie Curran and I had been out celebrating on Darwin Harbour aboard Sailing Yacht Nina Q1, a 63'Schooner. (I'd previously raced to Ambon Indonesia aboard Nina Q1; brag-brag winning Line Honours!) The following year, local kids were still chanting, "Ni-na Number One!-Ni-na Number One!" Oh-La-La, Debbie and I were hot to trot in Darwin, wearing silky, hired, frilly French laced-up bodice Can-Can outfits, complete with long blonde wigs, boa feathers and black seamed stockings thanks to dextrous use of a black marker pen whilst recumbent. It was hilarious and even funnier when we realised the pen was permanent as the hot nylon stockings came off. A touch too much sunshine is easy in Darwin.

Several other identical fun sailor outfits were worn. We both were glowing and hot yet snowing colourful tulle underneath. It took courage to shower and return to Can-Can-land wearing our sweaty silky outfits, but we did, for the sailing club show. We met many that night and later I noticed Errol in a photograph with a bit of his head chopped off. He was standing next to a guy whose t-shirt read, "Different Day, Same Sh**". I was such a prude back then that I even put a sticker over that guy's t-shirt in my photo album. Can you believe it?

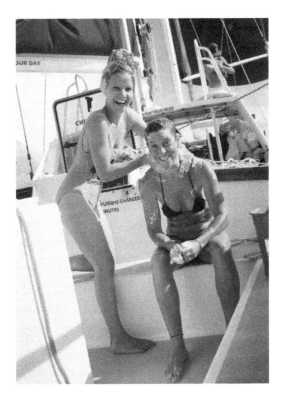

Aboard SY NINA washtime fun with Marcelle from Canada.

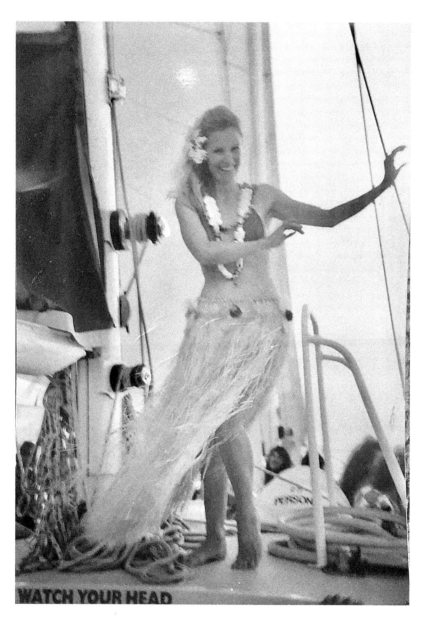

*I organised some popular twilight cruises
fundraising for a new sail.*

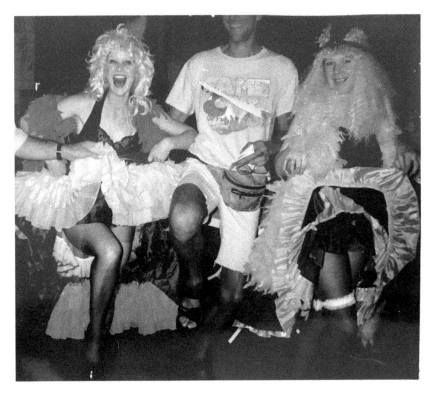

The covered Same Day shirt (Same day I met Errol)

This annual 1995 Darwin to Ambon Yacht race was my third to Indonesia, but my fourth international race, (I missed the 1992 and 1994 races as I was in French Polynesia). Pre-race excitement filled the air. I was hooked on racing internationally now, since being one of five different nationalities aboard 55' SY Australia Maid's 12-person crew and winning line honours in the Coral Sea Classic Race from Cairns to Port Moresby in Papua New Guinea.

This race was in preparation for the Darwin to Ambon Race. The advice was: learn to sail and choose a big boat for stability. Mission accomplished! Rene, the mother of the Mitchell Mob, had really encouraged me to proceed with this race. One son put fear and negativity into my mind that I didn't want to entertain. The cautionary comments pre-race weren't about falling overboard or Papua New Guinea, Land of the Unexpected, but were directed at the male crew and their potential to put me in a compromising position. Rene said, "Don't listen to naysayers—just go—you'll be fine and have a ball!" She was right! God love that woman!

A passage fee of AUD $500 per person was paid to contribute to costs and taxes. Four out of our 12 crew were women. I felt safe, followed instructions, and was a valued team member. Harnesses were rarely worn by any crew. Night-time on the Coral Sea was the first time I ever experienced seeing phosphorescence in the water! The beauty in this sea of glittering stars must be seen to be believed. It is caused by suspended living organisms producing light in response to external stimuli, surf, the vessel's wake, and fish movement.

Line Honours was exhilarating, and official check-in happened quickly at Port Moresby Yacht Club, (PNG). We were escorted across the road from the marina to the clubrooms and warned not to walk about by ourselves. The week before, a poor fellow had his arm axed off by some 'rascal'. It was particularly unsafe for fair-haired women. I soon flew back to work. The same year, 1991, on the return voyage to Darwin from Indonesia, against the weather, I was lucky to be aboard Line Honours winner 33-foot Darwin catamaran 'Electric Dreams' which we temporarily renamed 'Wet Dreams'! Voyages to Indonesia included 1991; Line Honours monohull; Nina QI Aluminium 63' schooner Darwin homeport, 1993; Summerwind 3 fibreglass 55' Siska-4 Sydney to Hobart racer from Adelaide, 1995; Balladier 55' ferrocement monohull Gove homeport. Each race was a vastly different experience, even though the course was the same, crews were from different walks of life, bringing varied skill sets and such a delightful tapestry of humanity.

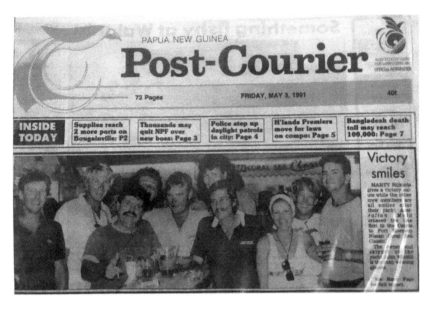

Newspaper photo: The crew of SY Australia Maid having won line honours in the Coral Sea Classic International Yacht Race (Cairns to Port Morseby, PNG). RIP Capt. Marty.

Looking back, we were extremely lucky nobody went overboard on any of these races in the Arafura Sea, although the winds were favourable and the seas mostly comfortable. Two to three-metre swells were usual on the course. Dolphins surfing them was always a bonus. Yes, I briefly experienced seasickness on the Coral Sea bound for PNG and found ways to avoid it, like keeping busy, not preparing carrots, curries nor fish-eye milkshakes, looking at the horizon or a fixed cloud, staying on deck for fresh air, spraying or bucketing saltwater from head to toe, breathing fast and deeply and briefly looking up at the sun. I desperately did not want this affliction, I sipped water and avoided time down below where the air was stuffy, hot and smelly (as the head was often in demand for a 12-person crew). These things made a world of difference for nausea. I had used anticholinergic, scopolamine in the form of a sticky dot behind the ear for sea sickness and Stugeron tablets but unfortunately, as a result, had slightly blurred vision, making needle threading a challenge for flag repairs. Not reading nor sewing helped! Other senses can mess with the brain's equilibrium. Years later, occasional bouts gave me empathy for others suffering mal de mer.

Seasickness was horrible when returning to Darwin against prevailing winds aboard the small lightweight catamaran Electric Dreams. Regardless, I was a trooper, making every effort to rid myself of nausea, staying hydrated, and mostly above deck when not asleep off watch. The sea was so rough and noisy on the hull, but sleep came easy as I was exhausted. Dry toast and crackers really helped. I occasionally sang *Fear Not*, a strongly religious song about God always being with us, especially in times of duress. The phrase "Fear not" is in the Bible 365 times! Incidentally, food supplies were very low, so not much for quarantine to check upon return to Australia. The other three crew members were outside downwind smokers and when the Darwin drug dog found something after much coaxing, we were all taken by surprise, but it had been planted as a reward exercise. There was a lesson born of both surprise and suspicion making me question how well I really knew that crew. No drugs on us!

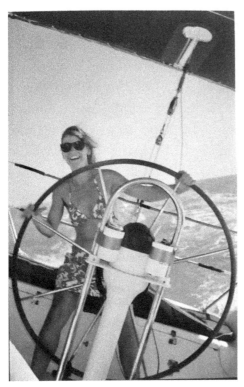

SY Mango Madness with Claire de Lune at the wheel.

Living away from my homeland has brought me to some difficult conversations. I've told Errol that if I was to go 'overboard' and I have been known to do that quite a bit in a different sense, please don't have search parties out looking endlessly. I believe once I'm gone from this world, my physical body won't matter and hopefully, others will remember me by my joyously free spirit.

Coming to Australia, the other, larger island down under, in the early 80s I

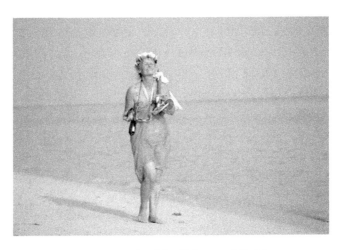

Leaning into the blissful, zen life I love.

136

saw beauty vast in contrast. I love Dorothea MacKellar's painting of words in **A Sunburnt Country** and have memorised this poem:

The love of field and coppice
Of green and shaded lanes,
Of ordered woods and gardens
Is running in your veins.
Strong love of grey-blue distance,
Brown streams and soft, dim skies
I know, but cannot share it,
My love is otherwise.
I love a sunburnt country,

A land of sweeping plains,
Of ragged mountain ranges,
Of droughts and flooding rains.
I love her far horizons,
I love her jewel-sea,
Her beauty and her terror
The wide brown land for me!

The stark white ring-barked forests,
All tragic to the moon,
The sapphire-misted mountains,
The hot gold hush of noon,
Green tangle of the brushes
Where lithe lianas coil,
And orchids deck the tree-tops,
And ferns the warm dark soil.

Core of my heart, my country!
Her pitiless blue sky,

When, sick at heart, around us
We see the cattle die
But then the grey clouds gather,
And we can bless again
The drumming of an army,
The steady soaking rain.

Core of my heart, my country!
Land of the rainbow gold,
For flood and fire and famine
She pays us back threefold.
Over the thirsty paddocks,
Watch, after many days,
The filmy veil of greenness
That thickens as we gaze ...

An opal-hearted country,
A wilful, lavish land
All you who have not loved her,
You will not understand
though Earth holds many splendours,
Wherever I may die,

I know to what brown country
My homing thoughts will fly.

Dorothea Mackellar

Preplanning for a yacht race included Debbie's completion of her master's degree in education in Melbourne. My mortgage in Christchurch was covered but I was a bit strapped for spending money until Debbie's holidaying Canadian friend came by for a spa after skiing one afternoon. Where she rented was cold, so I offered her my big bedroom and ensuite for less per week and she happily paid me 10 weeks in advance. Perfect. I just love a win-win! Mortgage payment and spending money: tick!

So, Errol officially met Debbie and me at the Darwin Sailing Club, with stunning Sally adorning his arm, by chance in the queue at the pre-Darwin to Ambon Indonesia race dinner, still wearing our can-can numbers. We thought they were a couple but later learned her husband knew she was an escort. They also had a yacht in Cullen Bay Marina. The queue for food was very long and small buffet pickings remained, so Errol suggested we all go elsewhere despite meal prepayment. I had 10 bucks on me and rehydrated on soup. Errol kindly paid for us all. Another night after visiting SY Nina Q1 in Cullen Bay Marina, Debbie and I paid a late visit to a lit-up MV Idlewise. Sally was sick in bed aboard, so it wasn't until the next time we met that she indicated she was looking for someone for Errol.

⚓ Debbie and I had our positions set aboard Bill Gibson's ferro monohull, "Balladier", a 55-foot ketch which was up on the hard stand having a DIY bottom job (antifouling) to glide through the Arafura Sea. Bill, rest his soul, was Commodore of Gove Yacht Club, sea savvy, and a gentleman. We competed in the racing category. Our passage was free, so with gratefulness, we assisted with hull work for new antifouling and prepared large vegetable-laden frozen stews and curries. These meals thawed quickly, were nutritious and easily reheated.

Debbie and I shared a bunk and happy hour treats at sundown. The 600 nautical mile race, north of Darwin was fanned by the Southeasterly trade winds that ancient seafarers had used for centuries when returning from Australian waters with sea cucumber or trepang for the Chinese market. It sometimes took days of doldrums to arrive up the long harbour to the excited villagers at the coastal town of Amahusu, Ambon Island in the Maluku Islands, Indonesia.

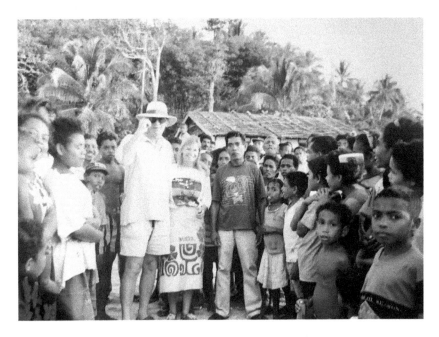

Welcomed ashore in Indonesia. We gave fuel for Meatimiarang's lighthouse, lots of clothing and overwhelmed the locals.

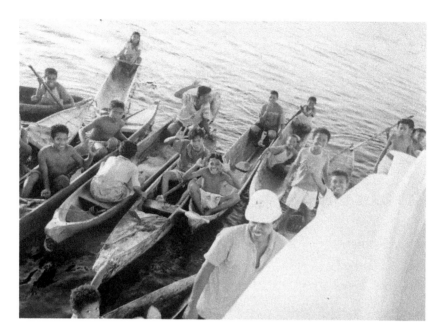

Indonesian Dug out canoes welcoming us.

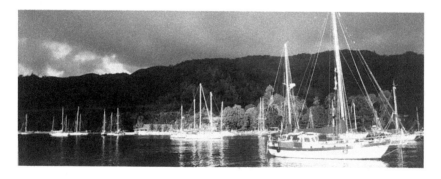

Yachts at Ambon Harbour, Maluku Regency, Indonesia.

With increasing popularity, some 130 (YES *one hundred and thirty!*) participating yachts from 11 different countries looked for a spot to anchor close to the food and entertainment. The wahrongs (little pop-up eating huts) along the beach were heavily stocked with beer. Those clever operators who kept Bintang beer chilled and flowing sold more. Tap water could cause diarrhoea. Added ice was optional! I love the spicy flavours of Asian food and was game enough to eat off the mobile Bakso carts without sickness. On subsequent visits, Errol dubbed these 'Death Carts'.

Local Ambonians really laid it on, honouring arrivals with the horn and flare, drums, whistles, extremely ornate costumes, and beautifully made-up women who had obviously practiced their traditional dances together for many months. Coloured flags adorned everything, mainly in red and white, which are Indonesia's national colours. Roadside fences were freshly painted. The gamelan drums clanged and tinkled, roosters loudly crowed any time of the day, and dogs barked, so many dogs, bus horns, and loud music; giggy-giggy boom-boom came out of everything that moved.

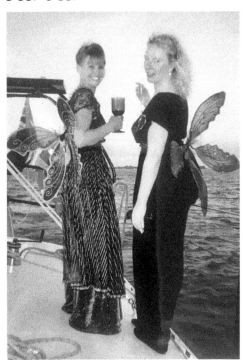

Social Butterflies.

Children in their smart, crisp white school blouses marched in lines to Keri Kanan Keri Kanan Left Right. The place was abuzz with excitement.

It was a laugh a minute when Debbie was around. She didn't want to abandon old Bill as all the rest of his crew had flown back to work in Darwin. That's what happens after the race, the crew leaves, and there's peace again for a solo captain. Debbie thought he needed crew.

They later experienced a rough voyage, a "hell ride", you could say, then were stuck in the doldrums, with no starter motor, nor radio, days going nowhere and at times, going backward with the tide. The onboard doctor was concerned about limited drinking water and let off a daytime flare. Debbie wasn't concerned. There was water and lots of warm beer, but it altered the way she observed this doctor who was panicky. Bastions of male supremacy, also around boats, have long disappeared as women are equally capable, running tight ships, sometimes intimidating male counterparts.

Competent, cool, and level-headed leadership is important at sea and on land. Errol's expertise always gave me confidence. He has always been a great fix-it-now captain with good diagnostic abilities too. He would've had Bill's starter motor going.

Something I remember well was hearing about a woman who had been stoned to death on that stony beach at Amahusu, Ambon Island one evening. My mind still cannot fathom the cruelty of human beings acting without mercy. I considered not including this information, but it was just as shocking to remember it all these years later. Bad things sometimes happen to good people. We only had to visit Ambon's War Cemetery to see the thousands of New Zealand and Australian servicemen buried there, who had travelled to help near neighbours fight the WWII Japanese invasion. Prayers with brothers and sisters set intention free yet anchors hearts and minds when busy or burdened, lightening the spirit. Locals remember in gratitude. Mastery of values, behaviours, meditation, the senses and the soul (and postures) bring us closer to the true essence of God and ourselves through concentration and the breath of life. This union or yoga brings peace and connection with worldwide family for our natural joy and passion in life. Indonesia's five principles are embraced in the Pancasila; nationalism, humanism, democracy, social prosperity and belief in one God.

Errol needed a new boat cook as French Agnes returned to Darwin. They were big shoes to fill but Debbie and I put our hands up. On my first morning underway aboard Idlewise, diesel fumes and the different roll caused nausea. A stink boat is what it is. I forgot Indonesian bread is very sweet, so the toast burned, leaving room for improvement. All these years later I appreciate my mum for the daily meals she cooked. We eat to live, not live to eat, but I try to maintain a healthy, balanced dietary intake. Often aboard, we have worked on 'tummy time'. It's very good for us to fast and then all food usually tastes better and is more appreciated.

⛴ In 1995, magnificent tall ships from all over the world gathered for the celebration of 50 years of independence from Dutch rule in Indonesia. This was another reason Debbie and I made the pact two years before to participate in this particular Darwin to Ambon race.

In Bali, Darwin race organiser, Angela, also came aboard Idlewise and voyaged to the Thousand Islands north of Jakarta. It's a chain of 342 islands stretching 45 kilometres north into the Java Sea at West Jakarta Bay. It was a truly majestic sight as tall ships gathered, their sails full, to race in the Madura Sea to Jakarta. I'd achieved my Radio Operator's Certificate in Darwin and assisted with twice daily alphabetical yacht high-frequency radio schedules for position reports to Ambon. We minimised chat, keeping the flow steady and clear like a precision time machine. Being the only spectator vessel, the request came to be the Tallship race start-boat opposite an imposing Indonesian warship, whose radio failed so we also ran these communications.

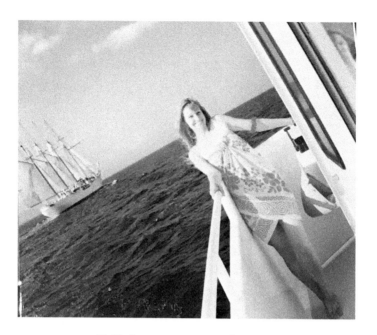

Tall ships race in Madura Sea

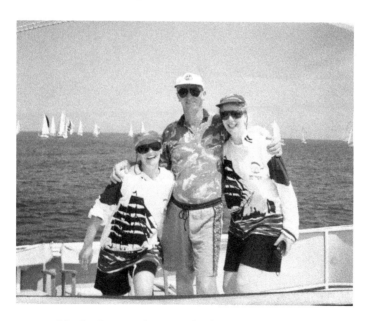

Yacht Races Thousand Islands, Indonesia.

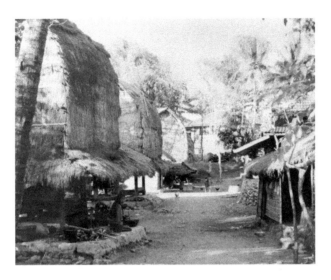

Lombok village visit.

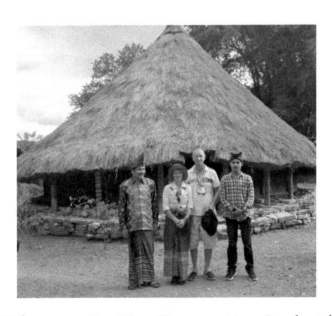

Kefamenanu, East Nusa Tenggara visit to Royals with sacrificial rooster ceremony. (Tour by English teacher Sipri)

Life really is a series of glorious opportunities, brilliantly disguised as impossible situations.

An invitation to attend the Tall Ship's Captain's formal dinner in Jakarta followed. It was assumed that we would already have appropriate garments aboard, so the pressure was on to impress. There was no gown in my backpack and my budget didn't extend to buying a gown and matching sparkly red shoes. Errol insisted on buying this gown. I had made a date with destiny, sparkling, glowing and holding his arm truly feeling special. He also bought himself an expensive suit that needed alteration and was to be collected the morning of the dinner.

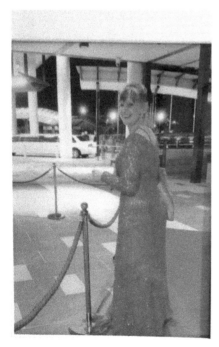

Matching red for Gold Coast University Hospital grand opening Sept 2013

Whilst grocery shopping in the mall where it had been altered, the bag containing the suit inadvertently was placed beside the counter and this wasn't noted until we were stuck in traffic later. We returned to find the mall's glass doors locked. Oh, dear! What now? We waved frantically at a cleaner mopping the floor. Hallelujah! He opened the door! In my very broken, but best pleading Indonesian, I explained and mimed the situation. He smiled, let us in, then led us through a kilometre of warren-like, narrow, back corridors to eventually find the security office. The relief upon seeing that suit bag on the desk was immense! We thanked them and surprised Debbie and our driver.

Time was short and traffic appalling but there was absolutely nothing we could do. We scrubbed up, changed, and scurried over to Tanjung Priok Naval Port to find the buses had already departed. An official Naval limousine magically appeared and took us to this special event on time. Police saluted our flagged vehicle with heavily tinted windows, clearing traffic so effectively. It was unbelievable. Upon arrival, our driver would not take payment and offered to take us home afterward giving us peace of mind. Great breakdowns can give us greater breakthroughs!

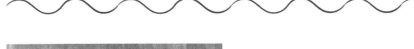

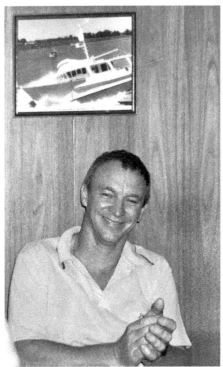

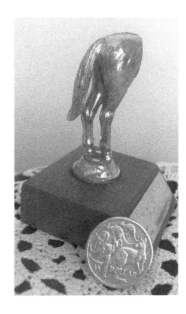

Young Errol clasping the much-coveted Horse's Arse trophy.

CHAPTER 9

THE WELL-SUITED GOOD CAPTAIN ERROL

$\smile$

Errol avoids wearing suits. At the red-carpeted entrance, I noted a white-uniformed official with a lot of gold braids on his shoulders and many medals on his chest. Having a small camera in my purse I suggested that we should go over and ask for a photograph with him and his wife. He delightfully obliged and we learned that he was the Chief of the Indonesian Navy, Admiral Tanto Kuswanto. This photograph, once enlarged and framed, was strategically placed next to another enlarged photograph of our friend, the Chief Minister of the Northern Territory, Australia, shaking hands with Indonesia's President Suharto. A third photograph connected the dots portraying Errol in his pilot captain's white shirt, complete with four gold striped epaulets and captain's cap, shaking hands with the NT chief minister and me, well covered in a long-sleeved white lace dress with an office wall map of Southeast Asia behind us. These photographs gave us immeasurable kudos for future travel throughout Indonesia. Many Indonesians boarding Idlewise knew who these powerful people were yet didn't know our connection.

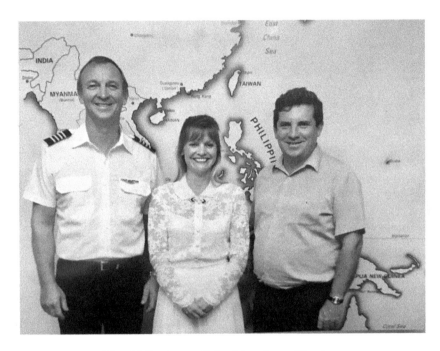

Chief Minister of the Northern Territory
at the time: Shane Stone QC

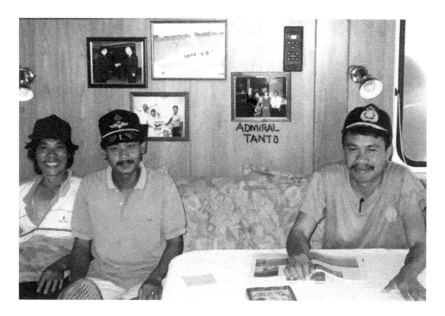

If I said "Photo for Jakarta" any cans (of beer) were removed. Cold drinks were a novelty. People in general throughout Southeast Asia are extremely polite.

The Tall Ships Captain's Gala Dinner event was the most opulent we had ever attended. Staff changed the candle-lit floral arrangement on our table four times. The food was delicious and so decorative. Intricately carved fruit was a true art form. Entertainment was world class and speeches were typically long. With true Indonesian integrity, our driver happily waited. At the completion of the evening, my long-sleeved, full-length red dress shone in the spotlights and driver 'Maday' found us in the crowd. We were overwhelmed to be treated like royalty. Police traffic controllers again saluted us. We insisted Maday keep our bonus gift for his family. Going the extra mile can take you far.

✝ After lots more great cruising, my holiday ended. There were responsibilities in NZ, hospital shifts to re-establish and I wanted to maintain my DC3 casual position as an air hostess. This was the dream job I cherished. As NZ winter ended, joy flights filled. I love big, radial engines, flying, big band swing music and serving champagne and hors-d'oeuvres in character 1940s uniform. I enjoyed giving the safety brief before take-off and landing and nostalgically painted boldly in white DC3-4ME on my dark green gabled roof for a buzz.

Pionair DC3 company later initiated a 10-day deluxe tour around NZ needing passengers to pay a $5000 fee. If I found a passenger, the hostess position was mine. Immediately I thought of Errol and his flying club friends. He was very keen, especially if I was to be the hostess. One of our hosties spoke German and she was chosen above me to translate for two Austrians. I let Errol know I wouldn't be on the trip and he replied, "Tell them I'm not coming unless you're there." Pionair decided to offer me the role of being an inside informant for passengers' gut feelings about every aspect of the trip. This was easy. I could relax and also be a passenger with Errol. Love was in the air around scenic New Zealand!

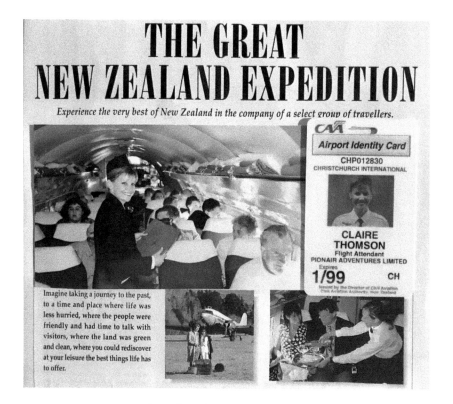

THE GREAT NEW ZEALAND EXPEDITION

Experience the very best of New Zealand in the company of a select group of travellers.

Imagine taking a journey to the past, to a time and place where life was less hurried, where the people were friendly and had time to talk with visitors, where the land was green and clean, where you could rediscover at your leisure the best things life has to offer.

Airport Identity Card

CHP012830
CHRISTCHURCH INTERNATIONAL

CLAIRE THOMSON
Flight Attendant
PIONAIR ADVENTURES LIMITED
Expires
1/99 CH

Claire Flight Attendant DC3

I sold my character house, farewelled the garden, returning to Darwin to be with Errol aboard Idlewise. For years, I told myself never to live with a man before marriage, pondering why buy the cow if you get the milk for free. It was not a perfect world. I had spent six years by myself. Life had become a dream come true, as Errol ticked my required qualities list. Love is a beautiful thing! I took time out from nursing and we just cruised, living the dream, doing Darwin to Ambon annual races as the radio communication vessel, boat work and Kimberley jaunts with lots and lots of laughs and fishing.

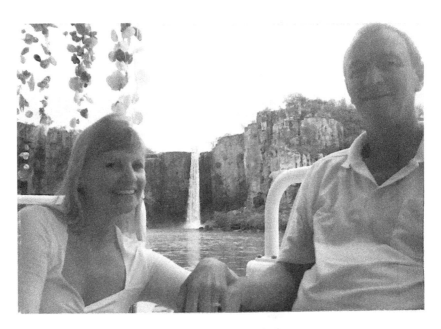

Amphitheatre Falls Berkeley River WA

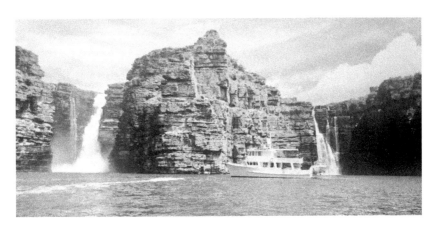

King George River and TSMV Idlewise

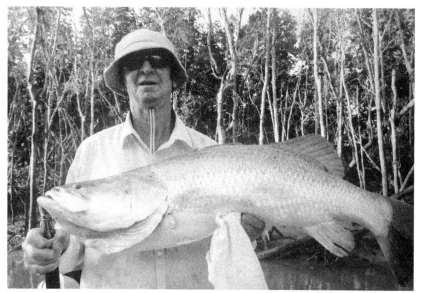

Happy man with a nice barramundi

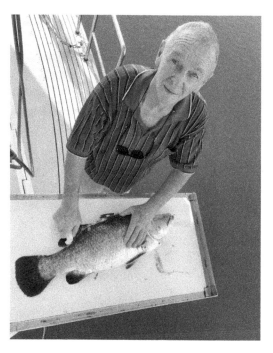

Filleting was sometimes a big job.

⚓ The 1998 Darwin to Ambon yacht race became the last for a decade as Indonesia was politically unstable and civil war broke out in the very Maluku Islands we had grown to love so much. Despite Muslim and Christian populations living peaceably together there for over 400 years, conflict resulted in massacres with hundreds of thousands displaced. The Australian government advised not to travel to Indonesia. I became an Australian citizen that year in Darwin. What better place to cruise than Australia's Kimberley paradise? Many friends we've had aboard say unequivocally this was the best holiday of their lives. In retrospect, we were lucky for no crocodile injuries. Errol being multi-skilled was good at luring crocs to his fishing line.

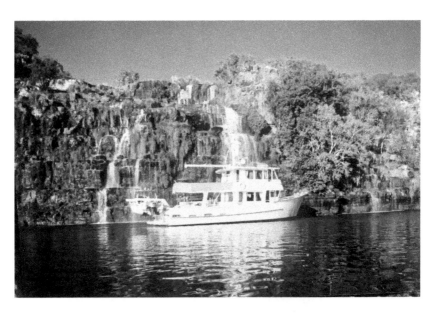

King's Cascades, Prince Regent River. This is also where American beauty Ginger Meadows was taken by a crocodile. I had a red heeler named after her in Darwin gifted by Sgt Boots.

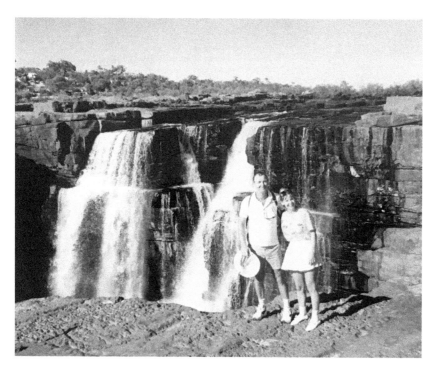

*King George Falls were always worth the
walk-up. Errol stumbled a lot.*

We both anticipated returning to friendly Indonesia. Political
stability returned and small international annual yacht races
departed initially from Darwin to Dili in East Timor and
Saumlaki in the Tanimbar Islands, Indonesia.

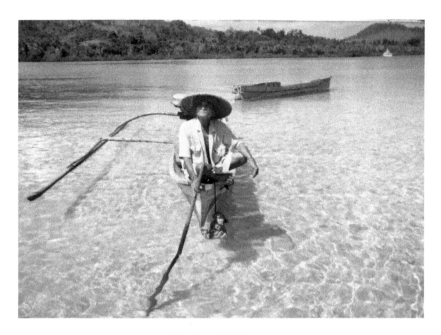

*A common sight: local fisherman in sampan
hat using coral as an anchor.*

⚓ The Kimberly WA, was also a majestic, rugged, remote, and exciting place to explore between Darwin's hub, voyaging north to Indonesia and beyond and south to family in Australia's Queensland (and over the Tasman Sea to NZ) then back up and over to God's other country: The Kimberley. This well-run route across the Joseph Bonaparte Gulf became very familiar. It took about 30 hours of travelling at nine knots nonstop for us. In town (Darwin), Errol tended to his list of daily maintenance and repair or techie jobs and generally, after two days back in port, I found work starting immediately as a casual nurse. It was great to contribute and sharpen my pencil. I was often welcomed back with, "How soon can you start? Tonight?" We kept a vehicle in both the NT and Queensland with friends or family.

I worked whatever shifts I could to accommodate staffing needs, and this was highly appreciated. Around shift work, I helped aboard. Our watches when doing overnight passages totally changed my attitude towards night duty. I learned to switch off and allow my body to sleep and rest as necessary when off duty. Errol already did this, stretching out for a siesta in the middle of the day especially. I loved returning to Darwin. We both loved the remote coastal Kimberley region, our backyard for 20 years, wishing we could spend the remainder of our lives there. I sang my own version of *Idlewise*; strong and white, clean and bright.Becoming Claire White, I saw more than 50 shades of love and light.

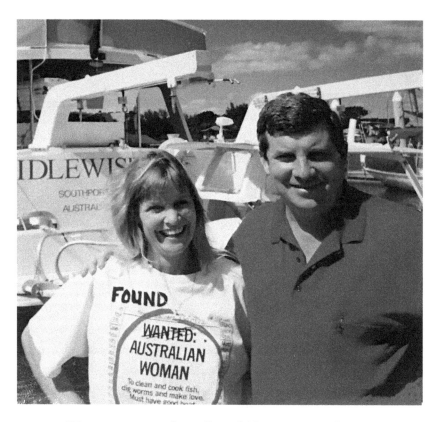

Honourary visit from friend Shane Stone after my
Australian citizenship was awarded by Mayor George Brown.

✝ **Errol, as in Flynn,** was 56, in Darwin from another voyage of Australia's remote Kimberley region in early 2002 when caring GP Dr. Barbara Allen referred him to Darwin Neurologist Jim Burrow. Errol had experienced unusual sickly-sweet smells, sweats, and headaches and his gait was a little different. Both arms swung on command, but one side appeared weaker. It was explained that normally, his patients weren't informed this early of Parkinson's Disease suspicion, but as we were soon leaving for Queensland by boat, he highly recommended we see another neurologist on arrival. We were in complete denial of this degenerative neurological diagnosis. I thought Errol was far too young and he didn't have the shakes I'd believed were synonymous with Parkinson's Disease. The most common symptoms are slowness, stiffness and shakes. We learned everybody's symptoms are different and there are other, worse neurological diseases.

In Queensland, familiar, basic neurological tests were repeated and another six months passed unmedicated. It became slowly, but progressively apparent that medical intervention and medications were needed when my assistance was required with fine motor skills, so pop domes replaced buttons and slot-head screws were replaced by Phillips heads. I helped him with belts, shoelaces and cutting steak. Thinking creatively reduces frustration.

Errol didn't want to be seen with the mask of Parkinson's, smiling on the inside, barely blinking and very straight or stone-faced outwardly, plus over salivating and dribbling. Dietary changes were needed, adding roughage, psyllium husks or oats, nuts and grains, more oral fluids, vitamin C, CQ10, fish oil and natural laxatives for regularity. Exercise, good hydration, and socialisation became equally important. Walking and cycling got us outside actively. Errol is also a good, sporadic, confident dancer, maintaining balance and poise.

We soaked up information and patiently waited 18 months between cruising destinations to see highly recommended movement specialist, neurologist and professor, Peter Silburn, in Brisbane. Errol had already sold his Cessna 210 JPL and didn't really miss flying at that time as we were busy refitting Restless M. Later he went halves in another Cessna 210, then sold out!

✚ In the discovery phase of Parkinson's Disease, we attended some Parkinson's group meetings held on the Gold Coast and saw a lot of people with different symptoms at varying stages of the disease. This was when we first heard of deep brain stimulation surgery. Errol proactively began drinking first milk (AKA liquid gold to midwives) although not human, but bovine colostrum, believing it had benefits.

We flew to Sydney for cutting-edge stem cell treatment, using cells separated from Errol's own spare abdominal and chest fat, which was sourced through liposuction, centrifuged, further separated by technicians and the syringe loaded with estimated millions of what were thought to be viable, concentrated stem cells, was then diluted in transportation saline and simply reinjected intravenously.

At a cost, two spare vials of Errol's stem cells were stored in liquid nitrogen in Sydney. Notably, his sore knees and lower back felt significantly better after the treatment, so he returned after a couple of years for round two of stem cells, but the count is still out re P.D. and neurologists killed off the placebo effect, saying any new brain cells eventually become 'Parkinsonised'. He offered his brain to Neurosciences Queensland for post-mortem research.

Neurologists were sceptical from the outset. They have never said, "Don't do it!" but advised a lot of money can change hands for little significant change. I didn't accompany Errol on that second trip to Sydney and was concerned for his safety travelling alone, as it became apparent that Parkinson's affected his movement and fine motor skills. He left his wallet in the taxi and got it back!

We adjusted to being moored at Hope Harbour and took on a massive project refitting 80-foot Restless M on the maintenance jetty. Idlewise sold. Parkinson's, as expected, continued. Errol saw another stem cell specialist in Southport, had hair follicle samples sent and began daily subcutaneous human growth hormone injections for the best part of a year, learning to self-inject. He visited an alternative Chinese Doctor in Burleigh adding also to his retirement fund and feeling good about the treatments. We continued to treat the symptoms that most affected his quality of life. "Remember sleep is your best friend," Prof Silburn said. In boating, fishing, cycling or doing what he loved most, dopamine and feel-good hormones were optimised.

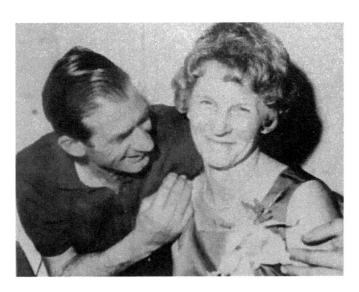

Keith and Nan White resting in peace now.

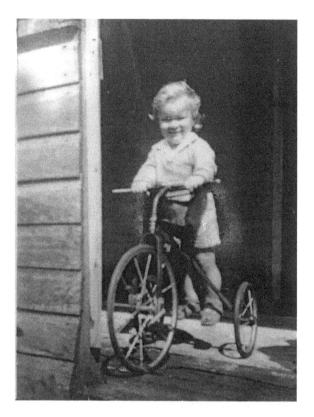

Errol aged two.

Errol is the second-born child of six. He was born near the end of World War II (Oct 1945). The war majorly influenced his parent's relationship. His father, Keith White, of Greek heritage and an armorer, was sent to Darwin and Bachelor with the Royal Australian Air Force. Smoking and cleaning inside large mustard gas storage tanks detrimentally affected his lungs and he later needed home oxygen. He was much younger than he told his wife and was granted early release from service on compassionate grounds for Errol's birth. Errol's biological father Ken came from the Bungawalbin area and was in the Australian Army Supply Chain, carrying the bullets and anything else required.

Meeting Ken and Agnes Gill (both RIP) and their family while we refitted Restless M meant a lot to us both. They have a strong resemblance.

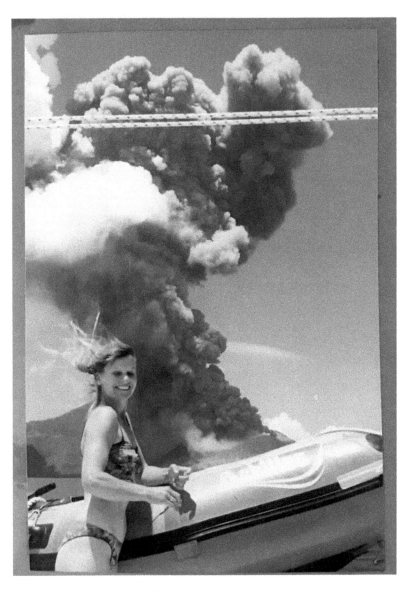

Near Rabaul 1996. We anchored on the Kokapo side of the harbour to avoid fine dust and enjoyed the nightshow fireworks.

164

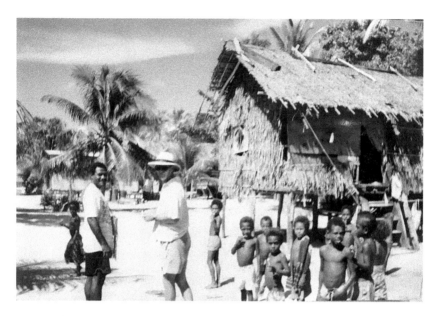

Sharing songs, maps, and flags at school. St John's First Aid equipment, tennis balls, footballs, pens, books, and blow-up globes were especially well received.

His parents worked on dairy farms in Camden, then in the Northern Rivers area. Keith and Ken did not know their own fathers. Errol says he and his brother could have easily been taken to a Catholic orphanage, but there was family understanding. His mother was also a very hard worker. Errol and his older brother were often sent from the family farm with grandparents at Bungawalbin, to stay with various aunties while their parents worked away. Times may have been tough, but they never felt unloved. The mixed farm was right on the floodplains of Sandy Creek. They milked before and after school, rounding cows on horseback, sometimes riding to school, or biking about four to five km. Errol didn't own a toothbrush until he was a teenager and first wore shoes when he went to secondary school. Chemical exposure is now proven to cause Parkinson's. Errol has used a myriad of chemicals over the years, often without any protection for his skin.

The family moved from Corakai to Burleigh Heads, Queensland, and Errol attended the Southport State High School, securing his first weekend job at 14, pumping gas at Burleigh Heads. The mechanic took him under his wing and taught him. He received his driver's license at age 16, having been told to just drive around the block while his father and the local policeman had a yarn.

Errol and his schoolmate, Wayne, worked in the E.S. and A. (England, Scotland and Australia) bank at Burleigh Heads and Southport. He became a relief officer in Cairns. From there, he went to Ayr and from Ayr to Brisbane, working in the staff department (equivalent to human relations). He was documented as an 'Officer with Outstanding Potential'. He married at almost 20, lived at Camp Hill in Brisbane and had three beautiful daughters. Whilst working in the bank, he bought a truck—an International SF 174. He had a driver but needed to do repairs and maintenance himself at night, so he bought another truck.

It became progressively more difficult to maintain his bank job and run the truck business, so he found a job in Brisbane for a year with the trucks, which led to a big concrete job offer. He left the bank, bought two more trucks and agitators, bought three tip trucks, then sold the agitators. He worked for the Department of Main Roads on a tender basis, did his own office work and took the tippers out to Winton, carting gravel on the Winton to Longreach Road. He lived in main road camps intermittently for about a year with 15 men on the job and meals for only 10, so he said he learned to eat fast.

The family moved to Longreach but missed Brisbane, so they moved from Longreach to the Gold Coast, having sold the trucking business. Errol then worked with his school friend, Wayne, initially at Labrador Park ripening bananas, having bought a share from Wayne's brother. They bought land on Brisbane Road, built the original shed and formed South Queensland Banana Ripeners PTY LTD. Wayne did the daily market run and Errol supplied the Gold Coast shops with bananas and lettuce. Banana boxes were hand lifted. Forklifts came later. They worked long hours and weekends with no paid holidays, sick pay, or superannuation. Cars and fuel perks came later. The company bought an empty shop and turned it into a hugely successful fresh produce market at Ashmore. A good offer came so it was sold.

⚓ TRAINS, BOATS, AND AEROPLANES

Errol's first boat was the Albert 2, a 24-foot Hartley powerboat, then came Reef Gypsy, a 25-foot Bertram, Tanveral, named after his 3 daughters, was a 42-foot Bristol built in India, then Tanveral, a 32-foot Randall, was set up as a game boat. He loved game fishing and sold the Randall keeping the name. Then he bought the twin screw motor vessel Idlewise in 1984, a 65-foot steel monohull one-off carvel-designed hull built in a paddock on the Shoalhaven River at Nowra near Sydney and launched in 1978.

He added a wheelhouse after removing the flybridge in about 1989. Tanveral 2 was a custom-built 24-foot Stessl tri-hull, followed by purpose-built Blackfin 30-footer "Tanveral 3". Both were for game fishing and often towed behind Idlewise, taking family and many friends on unforgettable voyages. Generosity extended to ensuring passengers needed a holiday after activity-packed travels aboard.

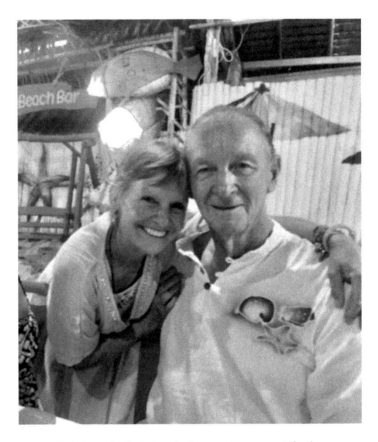

We loved The Beach Bar at Panwa, Phuket Thailand. Yes! I painted Errol's shirt.

Then Errol bought his first aircraft, SFS Cessna 182 RG (Retractable Landing Gear). In 1988, Errol took TSMV Idlewise to Coffs Harbour, tied up in the marina and booked in with the Aero Club Flying School. He was told, "We'll teach you to fly, but we won't teach you to fly 'that' as it's too fast!" He began, like everyone, in the smaller Cessna 152 focusing night and day on learning to fly.

From not knowing which side of the training aircraft's dual-controlled cockpit to sit in and barely being able to even keep a straight line on the taxiway, until he flew solo, took 10 days. After one month of daily flying on cross-country sorties, well outside the training area with his instructor, now endorsed in his 182, he flew back to Southport solo with his unrestricted pilot's licence. He remembers that great feeling of accomplishment well.

He later gave himself a fright switching off the autopilot to turn from the cloud, losing control and momentarily flying inverted in the cloud. Thankfully, he soon regained control from a downward spiral, prompting Instrument Flight Rating (IFR) training at Innisfail to fly through the cloud and at night. Biannual IFR endorsements were completed in Mudgee, New South Wales. The next aircraft was a Cessna 210 call sign JPL, a pressurised turbo-charged, airconditioned, six-seater with de-icing on the wings, windscreen and tailplane. Errol has always said that learning to fly is one of his greatest life achievements. He feels pleased and proud that one of his six grandchildren has taken up this skill as a profession. We remain members of the Southport Flying Club. He is hailed as a particularly good pilot. It is said that every landing you walk away from is a good one.

Errol was involved in the design, building and funding of the Gold Coast Game Fish Club. We held our wedding reception there. He volunteered with the Coastguard for a couple of years and achieved his radio operator's license and of course, the required first aid courses.

He also has a passion for collecting cars and tinkered with Morris Minors. These tallied 14 at one time, including one red Ute with a teak deck and buffed stainless-steel exhaust going up the cabin side (Incidentally, my first car was a Morris 8 Series E and he happily located another engine to replace its cracked head.)

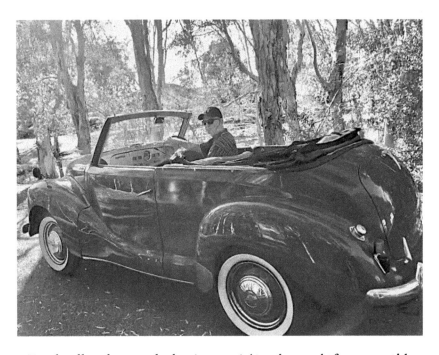

Errol still tinkers with the Austin A40 column shift convertible.

In life, it's also good to remember those who 'dug the well' getting things started and off the ground.

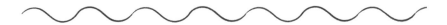

CHAPTER 10
DREAM IT–BECOME IT!

Just Plain Lucky is what I called the Cessna 210 aircraft with callsign JPL. Recognising local landmarks from the air was rewarding. Gliding taught me to regularly identify the safest place for an emergency landing. The coast of Queensland has many islands and with annual Southport Flying Club Safaris, Errol also circumnavigated Papua New Guinea before we cruised around by boat for over two years. This fulfilled his vision of visiting Sorong, Manokwari, Jayapura, Vanimo, Wewak, Blupblup Island, where we were robbed, Kar Kar Island, Madang, out to Manus Island in the Bismarck Sea, where we were robbed again despite my sign: "Itambu; snek e likem kai-kai yu!" translating to, "Keep off! Beware of hungry snake!", and around the top of New Hanover down to Kavieng on the Northeastern tip back through New Ireland and around to Rabaul along New Britain, diving at Kimbi, Umboi Island where 'Elvis Lives' is carved into a coconut trunk, on to Finschhafen, Tufi, Goodenough Island and down to Milne Bay's Aloutau, Samurai Island along the

Louisiade Archipelago to Bagaman Island, clearing customs and quarantine in Cairns, Australia. Cruisers visiting PNG were rare back then. Many canoes visited us by day, often with fruit and I enjoyed learning Pidgin English. Locals guarded MV Idlewise, often with a bow and arrows if we were ashore by night. We preferred staying home. Despite their 'rascals', we felt safe.

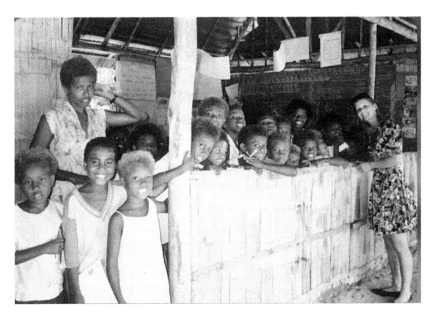

Many primary schools were visited with gifts of books, pens, maps, first aid equipment, balls, balloons, caps, flags skipping ropes, etc Songs and smiles were shared.

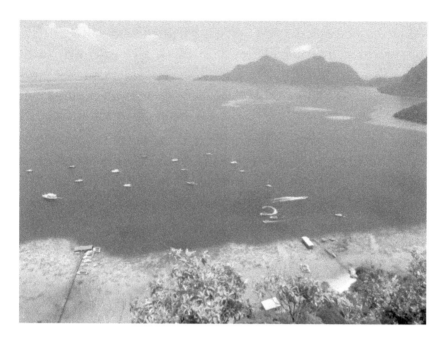

*Spectacular Boyheydulang Island near
Semporna, Sabah Malaysia.*

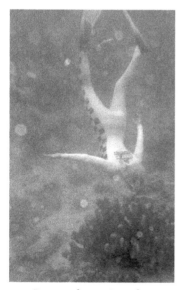

*Racey diver Sipidan
Island, Sabah Malaysia.*

We dropped anchor out wide at Osprey Reef Queensland, Australia, where 275-foot glamour megayacht, White Rabbit, was anchored. A 47-foot Sea Ranger named 'Funrey' was also at anchor. We chatted by radio, commenting light-heartedly about us poor people being over in the wood heap and an invitation to

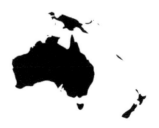

173

dinner for homemade pasta and garden salad soon followed. The idea of a garden salad had me salivating. To this day, I gratefully remember the beautiful flavours of coriander, cucumber, and mandarins inside that salad.

Not everything goes to plan for mice and man and upon our arrival in their dinghy, in case Coastwatch flew over, stepping aboard, Errol slipped, putting his tooth through his bottom lip, requiring ice, and dry clothes. Completing the boat tour at the engine room, once reassured there were no cameras nor second exit, I followed the captain's 'naked' rule for entry, for a laugh, discreetly wrapped in a towel, my garments were finger-twirled in view of our surprised captains! What a pair! I side shake my head at myself in disbelief, as we'd only just met! Truly, it was hilarious, and they've dined out many times on that introductory story too. I'm comfortable in my skin and don't mind being the laughingstock.

The following year, we covered muddy Irian Jaya, now known as West Papua, frightening ululating women who, upon seeing us, grabbed their children and ran for the higher ground above their huts, while their menfolk hurriedly retrieved bows and arrows from dug-out canoes along the bank. It didn't hold the same beauty as the Northern side. They also faced startling poverty. We gave away gifted clothing and toys outgrown by our own grandkids and family. We were offered 'kakup' (barramundi) crocodile and venison from muddy dugout canoes.

⚓ Errol has always enjoyed teaching others how to fish. He was my master guru and from the first moment he took me to the hotspot in the Little Moil River, N.T., I was addicted—hook, line, and sinker. Over 75 Bara in 1.5 hours, in fact, we lost count. It was all catch and release by memory that day. There were double hook-ups, and the fish were crazy on the bite. Frenzy fishing is an amazing phenomenon. They were absolutely on fire making me Barra Queen! We ate lots of fish we had caught providing plentiful protein and optimal Omega 3 for years.

We've always been super cautious around hooks, but the occasional one has gone into the back of a hand, through a finger, or into the leg. Believe me, you don't want to be hooked, least of all, to a flapping fish! So, we always make sure that anybody who's fishing with us wears a wide-brimmed hat, protective sunglasses, and footwear. First, free the fish from hooks. The safety uniform includes covering limbs to protect against sunburn and insect bites. Errol was generous with fishermen while we travelled, giving out lures and fishing line. He does enjoy setting a young person up with a rod and reel, including our own grandchildren who, at age one, had a custom-made fishing rod personalised with their own name, secured on special brackets above their beds, promoting dream building, natural curiosity, and delayed gratification.

"Give a man a fish and you feed him for a day. Teach a man to fish and you feed him for a lifetime." Lao Tzu

Errol said his three daughters married well. They all had a pigeon pair and all grandchildren enjoyed time well spent aboard and ashore with us over the years, sometimes without parents. The next generation has now come. Being involved with friends and family babies is so lovely and special. We can't get enough! The love we give just multiplies and our hearts overflow unconditionally.

Having good quality, respectful relationships, guarding our emotional and physical health against stress, while living true to ourselves, is a great blessing. Sharing love allows bonding and the gifts of knowledge, wisdom, hope and connection. Errol has always been an avid reader, especially enjoying crime investigation, espionage, murder and mayhem thrillers. He often reads several books simultaneously. He still enjoys tinkering with cars, watching racing and rugby league, each year picking his winners. He enjoys old cowboy movies, nature documentaries, and history.

Music. Yes, he's a fan of two types of music: country and western and has a good singing voice. He's also a spontaneous dancer, especially in the galley. He can crack a mean whip and was a good horserider in his day.

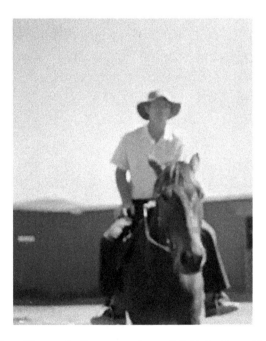

In Errol's cattle farming days. (BC; before Claire)

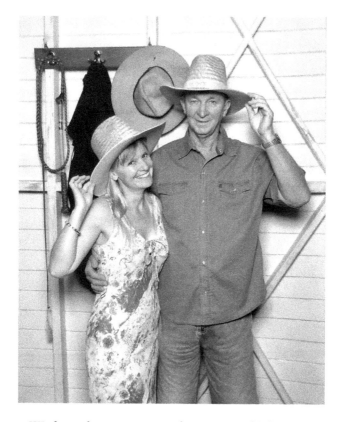

We love this country and our way of life. Yeeha!

He loves boating, above all.

⚓ In 2002, we bought the monohull motor yacht Restless M, a Bond Eighty, and spent another five to six years transforming her from a sow's ear to a silk purse, with time, effort, and money. Errol had a great vision over the years and seized opportunities as they came his way. He's proactive and has always been a doer, not a talker. This is why he has been so successful. He worked hard. His work and play ethic is exceptionally good. He remained open to possibilities, has always been fair in business, leaving a little for the next person, and paid his bills on time. He's also made some lucky

177

choices and has no regrets. He did the best with what he had at the time, honours effort for payment, had no entitlement expectations from parents nor government, ran with opportunities, took some risks and we have reaped the benefits. I'm so happy he found me.

We all know of people who just retire to find something unexpected happens and their life takes a turn, changing their retirement dreams entirely. TIP: examine what is on your own bucket list, clear any negatives or anything that weighs you down, and live life to the fullest. We all know life is not a dress rehearsal and we are worthy to fall in love with being the best version of ourselves with patience, compassion, and respect for our own journey.

Transmutation: grapes must be crushed to make wine. Diamonds form under pressure. Olives are pressed to release oil. Seeds grow in darkness. Whenever you feel crushed, under pressure, pressed, or in darkness, you're in a powerful place of transformation and transmutation. Trust the process! – Lalah Deli

---

I bargained with God for just a season aboard for all Errol's labour's reward. Twenty-seven years full-time was a good season! Once Restless M was up to a standard where we could go out cruising, we headed off to the white, sandy, coral-fringed jewel of Capricornia; Lady Musgrave Island in the Bunker Group of the Capricorn Coast Queensland, for her maiden voyage and the lagoon filled with friends. Each year, we headed a little further north again and then back over to Western Australia. Our days were filled with cruising, fishing, filleting, fun exploring, beaches and waterfalls. It was pure heaven on a stick.

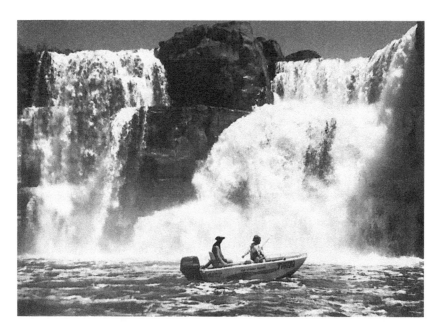

Casuarina Falls, Berkeley River WA

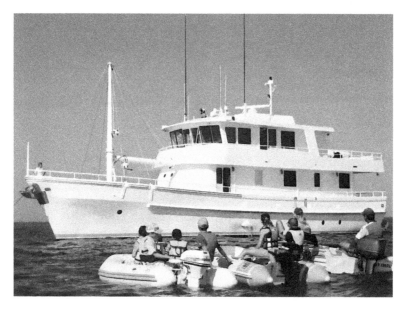

Lady Musgrave lagoon full of friends and fun.

We loved cruising back in the very windy, strong currents of the Torres Strait Islands for a couple of years around at least 274 islands; Thursday, Horn, Prince of Wales, Booby, Friday, Tuesday and Wednesday Is, Mt Ernest, Aureed, Campbell, Warraber, Poruma (Coconut Is), York, Yam, Darnley, Dalrymple, Stephens, Mer, (AKA Murray) right up close to PNG, Boigu and Saibai Islands with great friends Les and Jill (first met in Gove's Inverell Bay) of M.V. 'Fiddler 5' and met Les' missionary schoolfriend of Cat 'Another Angel' up there. It was not for the faint-hearted. Mum (Nan) White, my parents, Joe and Ross, also toured here with us.

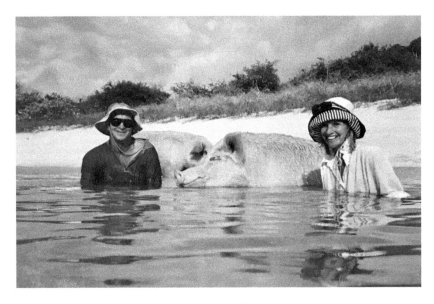

Swimming with the friendly sole inhabitants of
Campbell Island, Torres Straits, Australia

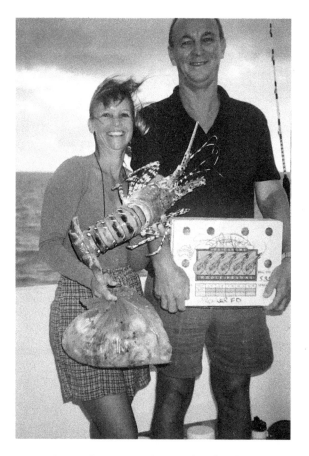

We are always happy and grateful for fresh seafood.

Honestly, these were some of the best years of our lives, living in Heaven on Earth off fresh fish, prawns and crayfish galore, white sandy beaches and friendly smiling islanders.

One did remind us, whilst cutting up a turtle for a feast, that it wasn't very long ago we 'whities' were on the menu! The Torres Strait Islands hold a special place in my heart. Seaman Dan (RIP) added to that with his special island music. I love the vibrancy, the easy and steady manner of the people with their colourful, relaxed rubber-time, Melanesian smiling nature and values.

A side story of perspective... My second-born Kiwi nephew Adam, when about six years old (delivered into this world by midwife me!) looking puzzled asked, "Auntie Claire, you live on a boat, don't you?"

"Yes!" I said adding, "You already know that Adam. You've been aboard and have seen lots of photos. Why do you ask me this?"

His response was, "Well, Gran said you live in a 'gin-palace'!" I understood his bewilderment! I have felt like a Queen and one's home is one's castle. Also, I'm rather partial to an occasional gin and tonic.

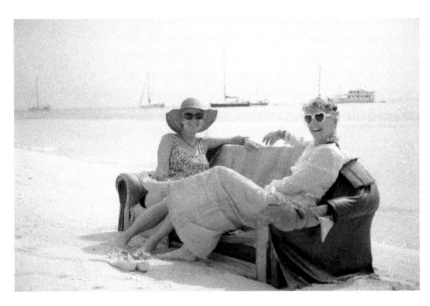

'On the Couch with Claire' *Girlfriend Melian, met in Kimberleys, cruised and posed with me on beautiful Ketawai Island, Indonesia. We've shared many sundowners.*

In vastly diverse cultures, surrounded by castles in Europe, we supported two grandsons in Junior and then Open Sailing World Titles in Ireland, Italy, and Germany, catching up with old friends and making many new ones. We saw my N.Z housemate and totally surprised ourselves and holidaying Aussies from Mount Tamborine QLD in Yorkshire and in Scotland joined Kimberley friends. I was thrilled Errol had this taste of Europe and knew more air travel would be on our horizons when our boating phase ended. Meanwhile, knowing the world is small can be comforting.

✚ The following year, in April 2013, we were ready, so we booked for Errol's deep brain stimulation (DBS) surgery. Professor Silburn said this was proven to be more effective against Parkinson's progression the earlier attended. We read up on the frightening list of potential complications and expected outcomes, weighing up the pros and cons. Primarily, though, we went on the advice of the neurologists: the sooner the better for the best long-term results and a 92% to 95% success rate. We read about the associated risks, that there would be a period of fine-tuning after the device was turned on and a little about the honeymoon phase post-operatively when Errol would likely feel elated. He was in good shape physically and mentally for surgery. The occupational therapist filmed his ability to side-click heels not quite at hip height, with both his feet together in the air. Thus, he was in fine form preoperatively, also being in the habit of easily cycling 15 kilometres per day around Hope Island.

Brain surgery postponement was requested by daughters as they were overseas. No problem. There were some claustrophobia concerns with the surgical halo to deal with. Claustrophobia has come and gone over the years. We have dived on a Mitchell Bomber at 80 feet in Madang, PNG and sat in the armed cockpit with no problem, and maintenance sometimes dictated crawling into small spaces for us both! Yet, one time in Darwin, pre-DBS, he felt confined with a panic attack coming on, so bolted from the MRI machine, grey and sweaty, refusing to return! Somehow, we slipped through the DBS psychologist's check net regarding that anxiety.

Taking the leap of faith, wires were inserted into Errol's movement regulation centre (targeting the Sub Thalamic Nucleus). In P.D., the progressive loss of dopaminergic neurones causes an alteration and abnormal firing pattern in the Sub Thalamic Nucleus. Deep Brain Stimulation modulates STN firing, helping motor and non-motor disabilities. The connecting wires are just below the skin and extend from the chest computer up the side of his neck behind his right ear for insertion through the skull. During deep brain surgery,

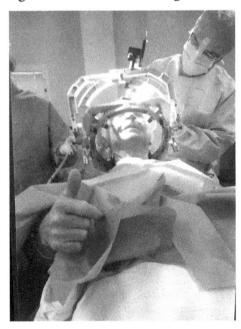

the anaesthetist kindly sent me a photograph of Errol awake, giving a thumbs up under the big halo-framed structure, which was bolted to Errol and to the operating table to prevent any head movement during surgery. His temporary consciousness was critical, allowing neurological tests to be performed and ensuring wires were in the exact (sweet) spot within the STN prior to cementing them into position.

Errol awake during brain surgery giving thumbs up.

Seeing haloed Errol awake during brain surgery was very emotional for me but it was good to know that he was doing fine and in the best of hands.

He woke up in intensive care telling me he had finished the book.

"What book?" I asked, knowing he is an avid reader and that he hadn't been reading.

"You know, writing!" he said. "That book I've been writing all these years in my sleep." I knew about this, as many mornings he had woken to say how tired he felt from being busy writing another chapter in his sleep overnight, yet he didn't even know the subject matter, despite me asking at various times.

The next morning, he was transferred to the ward, declaring upon my arrival, "Guess what?"

"What?" I asked

He continued brightly, "I have a name for the book!"

It's called "Who's in Charge, My Brain or Me? and YOU are going to write it!" This did blow me away at the time, but I took it in my stride, knowing it was possible.

✛ My guesthouse was only about 500 metres away. A few nights after his brain surgery, early in the morning I heard a rat-a-tat-tat on my bedroom window. I quickly let him in. It was particularly cold outside. He was cold to the touch despite his tracksuit and was smiling like a Cheshire cat, incredibly pleased with himself. A beanie covered his bandaged head. I warmed him up and asked him for reassurance that the staff knew his whereabouts.

"Well, sort of," he said. "They don't know exactly where I am. I just told them I was going for a walk."

They didn't know he'd left the hospital. He began telling me how he had snuck out along the corridor, hiding in each room's entrance alcove, and tippy-toeing, like the *Pink Panther*, between other patient's doorways along the corridor. This indicated that he knew exactly what he was doing surreptitiously. In the main foyer were big glass-locked front doors. Bingo! He located the green button behind the pot plant exiting to freedom.

He was still laughing when the hospital staff rang looking for him. They had sent wardsmen out into the park opposite the hospital searching, asked if he was ok and if he would please come back! Errol thought it was quite funny, men with torches wearing white coats out calling, "Mr. White-Mr. White, are you all right?". We went straight back, with nurse me chastising him! It was no honeymoon, but he felt pretty good about himself.

The following morning, he did say, "This isn't a prison, you know!" This attitude towards hospitals has continued. Professor Peter Silburn and Surgeon Doctor Terry Coyne visited post-operatively, adjusting his Deep Brain Stimulator with their programming device. He felt great and had ward leave before discharging. His confronting Frankenstein-ish staples were removed. He came home and then the fun really began.

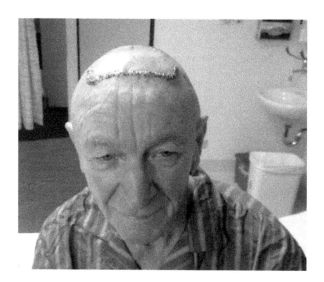

Errol's best Frankenstein likeness.

Incremental tune-ups were via telephone with the DBS nurse guiding him. He was compliant and attuned to his walking especially. Things gradually began to deteriorate. Speech became extremely fast and pressured with frothing at the mouth as a result. He had racing thoughts. Ideas galore. In fact, he thought he had superpowers because everything he seemed to think came true, he believed he had the Midas touch, everything he did was what he wanted, and really, he could jump tall buildings, leap in bounds over people, and get things done.

The trouble was that all the extra jobs weren't happening at his desired speed. He was trying to manage about 10 different teams and began getting frustrated with people when delayed. He was more irritable and his explanation for temper and intolerance was that his already short wick had been halved in surgery. He showed some argumentative traits that were not normal in his nature. The guys working for us witnessed this and tried to intervene when he stepped aboard another vessel to sort the problematic guy out. It was obvious I had my hands very full, and that Errol's mind was equally as loaded. Over time, things did settle.

We took Restless M over to Bum's Bay, Gold Coast. The Water Police stopped us in our dinghy one night when called about Errol's hospitalised mother. Errol began a disagreement with them over a navigation white light. His attitude almost caused a fine, but we got a warning instead to get it fixed. Done. These arguments started to crack me. I reduced my working hours to casual for increased flexibility and time with Errol.

He started two other businesses called Kimberly Tagalong Tours and Pedal Cars Australia. These ideas were all well and good, but without consultation with anyone else and there were no feasibility business studies conducted. He was offended when family members questioned him about why he would want to do that at his stage in life, answering, "Because I can. Don't you think I can?" He portrayed the 'I'll show you' trait.

Meanwhile, Errol's phenomenal powers of prolonged prediction regarding who would win the football began to show cracks. Initially, he had told everyone his experience was like the movie *Phenomenon*, and that his brain was going 100 miles an hour. He was functioning at an extremely elevated level, not sleeping much and forgetting simple things like drinking and tact. His filters fell off. He sometimes stepped beyond OK boundaries too.

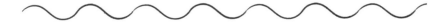

CHAPTER 11

CRASH AND BURN? HELL NO!

Errol purchased an Austin Devon 40 convertible on Gumtree as a promotional vehicle for his newly formed pedal car company. Being new to the online purchase process, he didn't know the car was near Sydney, NSW, so he then organised its transportation to Queensland. The vehicle meanwhile was uploaded onto the transportation truck prior to being started. Errol wanted to start it up, so he climbed onto the truck deck. The old Austin started but had major issues and didn't run sweet. His mood turned dark thinking he was conned.

The Austin was transported without a problem. Errol was on a mission to take it to a family gathering in Brunswick Heads NSW the following month. He needed the tyres changed for pickup Saturday morning. On Wednesday or Thursday, the job wasn't done. Reassurance annoyed him when he went to collect the vehicle Saturday morning only to find it wasn't even in the job line-up as the reverse gear on the column shift couldn't be found, despite the guy knowing all about it on arrival. Annoyed, Errol re-parked it, getting offside with the owner of the business and with the young worker who was keen to finish up and leave. There was swearing. He was busy changing other tyres and packing up soon to go home. Errol began the job himself. His aggression resulted in him being sprayed in the face with some liquid. We guessed it was probably soapy water, used for checking tyres for air leaks. It stung his eyes, so he went next door into his own property at the Banana Ripeners to wash his face. He rang me distressed. He'd basically been assaulted. This was another red flag as it was out of character for Errol to be so provocative and get so wound up.

Errol's mother, rest her soul, was in the hospital with pneumonia a month after his brain surgery when he bought all the hospital florist's stock and argued to have the loaded trolly delivered to her. Mum was a real trooper, recovered, and had another five or six lives until age 94 when melanoma took her. He had treated his mother and her sisters to a 200km limousine rendezvous with more sisters joining in Casino from the Gold Coast. He gave them the time of their lives. He pleasantly brought his natural parents together for afternoon tea on that trip, just months after his brain surgery.

Errol had followed doctors' and nurses' advice and fine-tuned his device per telephone from Neuro-Sciences Queensland's office, using mobility as the gauge. Unfortunately, the parameters set were within a trigger zone for him for mania.

✝ A lot wasn't in alignment. Family issues easily blew out of proportion, and more than twice, he left a daughter's place angry. I was running around behind him, begging for understanding, mopping up the fallout and putting out fires. Intimidation extended to me. I soon wised up and stayed at my girlfriend's house, giving him an opportunity to reassess and see himself as the drama's common denominator. He decided he didn't need anyone and could do everything himself. Maybe he began with a good process but pulling the boat's large pantry apart, throwing out whatever had expired, soon went to custard, as cans and bottles were everywhere, over benches, and the carpet as well was in large containers. Then he moved to the next job. Self-care obviously was lacking. Clothes, chip bags and Coke cans were scattered around the boat. Tools, books and papers were strewn as if looking for something.

Errol admitted he stopped at Ballina, NSW to use the Return Serviceman's League's bathroom and with $10 in his pocket, knew he would turn it into $60, which he said he did. This was also concerning as Errol was never a gambler. Stressed, he even spoke of just disappearing off the planet entirely, taking the car somewhere and just not coming back, as relationships had deteriorated all around him. He was high and mighty, impulsive and very unpredictable. All these little clues were of great concern to the neurologists who had seen this pattern before. He refused to attend the neurologist's meeting which they changed to an earlier date, opting for his own boat trip on the Richmond River.

🔆 He wanted to buy and set up a flying park on the flats of the old family dairy farm, about three miles from Corakai, Northern NSW. He would put in the runway and pilots would buy a block of land, and build their own place and hanger. He wasn't concerned about the massive financial outlay for minimal return, headaches with CASA (Civil Aviation Safety Authority) the regulator, nor the site being on a known floodplain. Nearby Sandy Creek flows into Bungawalbin Creek which flows into the Richmond River and these flood from time to time.

Errol ran the proposal past his lifelong solicitor friend and was not happy about his ideas being thwarted. There was no feasibility study considered. I was horrified that he could do something like this when we didn't outright own our home (boat) yet, let alone start up other businesses on a whim, yet knew he understood success.

A plan to send two mental health workers to check on Errol was implemented. He was elated, thought of them as being school-aged, showed them around the boat, and rapidly gushed all the projects he had underway, certainly showing himself to be manic, with pressured speech, and a flight of thoughts. They also mentioned in their report that upon leaving, he had hugged them both and then clicked both his heels off the ground together on each side. This is something Errol has always done, but these girls didn't know that. They rang me afterward, agreeing he was quite manic and understanding our concerns. They sent their assessment to the mental health team who activated the next step to have him taken to hospital under the Mental Health Act to have his brain device downturned.

We encouraged him to make an appointment to have his DBS adjusted, but he wouldn't have a bar of that, saying he was, "Fine, thank you very much, just go!" Everything was falling apart around him, including his family, who felt intimidated. The psychiatrist had already experienced intimidation by Errol's pointer finger repeatedly and firmly downward tapping on his desk when making unhappy points. We decided something had to be done for his own safety. I went with two of his three available daughters to meet with his specialist team in Brisbane. We were armed assertively for action, proposing his device be turned down. If he didn't agree, the alternative was to have him taken into care so it could be tuned down before he sustained an injury or approached a crash-and-burn scenario. I knew withholding knowledge of his behaviours was not protecting, nor helping him now. I'd hidden some since we first met. Being gracious, kind, non-judgemental and compassionate is powerful, costs nothing, and can change someone's world, so can the truth and a paradigm shift. Aesop said, *"No act of kindness, no matter how small, is ever wasted."* True colours shine through, yet Errol didn't see us as his allies.

"Sailing under false colours" was once a common deception of pirates flying a friendly flag until closer to potential targets (other ships) without causing suspicion. When their pirate ship was alongside, true colours unfurled.

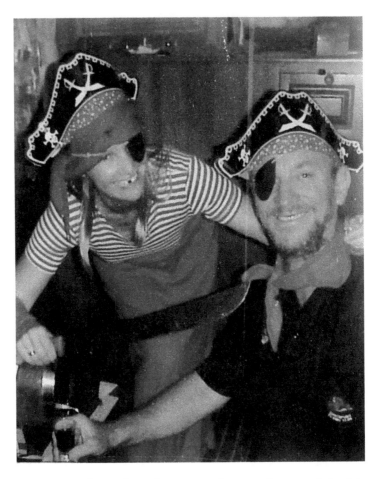

"There's so much good in the worst of us, and so much bad in the best of us, that it ill behooves any of us to find fault with the rest of us." James Truslow Adams. Remembering Jim Murphy who first taught me this verse modified, and highly recommended we cruise Borneo. RIP circumnavigator. Argh me heartie!

✚ Errol was taken to the old Gold Coast Hospital, not the newer Robina Hospital as was anticipated. I was rostered on the afternoon shift that day in the Emergency Department and was reallocated to work elsewhere as he awaited assessment there. He was not happy, especially with my part in it. He texted a few mates on his way in, saying he was in the back of a police car, Claire was behind this and had gone 'leso'. I was staying at a girlfriend's safe haven, bless her! His brother wanted to take him home but wasn't permitted. They didn't understand why. Errol felt all his rights had been taken and they had, for his own safety.

It was a very distressing time for us all. It was a Friday. The Medtronic Company's technician arrived wanting to check the brain stimulator device settings and immediately changed it. To this day, Errol calls him a liar for turning it down. He quickly went from being manic to zombie-like, unable to do much for himself. There was no coordinated plan from Neurosciences in Brisbane. An hour's drive was too far away for them, so frustrating for us. Errol dumped all the family and me, and all we could do was continue to work our unconditional love on him, be patient and wait for his improvement.

Errol was asked to hand in his firearm which he voluntarily did. He was offended by the police letter saying he was not a 'fit and proper person' to hold a licence because he was in the hospital under the Mental Health Act so, by law, could not hold the licence. Once his brain device was turned down, he was given the option to reapply for a gun licence. He didn't bother. He clung to the 'not a fit and proper person' statement though, ruminating over it and distressing himself unnecessarily.

He voiced that the neurologists were actively trying to organise to take over the world by implanting these brain devices, stating there's a book online titled *Murder by Medtronic*. It's there. He hasn't read it. Of great concern was that he also thought that he would be able to leave town and return to his high-functioning DBS setting by purchasing his own programmer like his specialist used.

Alexander Pope (1771) wrote:

Essay on Criticism

A little learning is a dang'rous thing. Drink deep, or taste not the Pierian spring; There shallow draughts intoxicate the brain and drinking largely sobers us again.

The psychologists were having a field day! I loved the coffee cup of one which read:

PRIORITIES: 1: My coffee 2: Your problems

Errol began to think that he knew a lot more about his own neurological disorder than he did. It was his body, after all. So, he decided, without any discussion, to buy his own deep brain stimulator programmer online. This was just part of the nightmare. It was posted from England to a daughter's house, and that's where it remained. Fortunately, the programmer was incompatible with his device anyway.

I tried reasoning with him by simply asking how he intended to use it. Believing in his own intelligence he said he could read the manual. I asked if he had 10 years of medical and specialist training as well. I reminded him when adjustments were made, he would sometimes go blind, questioning how he would do his own programming in some remote area without sight. Did he think I would simply follow instructions and assist? (The blind leading the blind!) I was totally against it! The programmer did not come aboard nor did it go on the black market endangering another.

He received a letter from the Senior Legal Counsel Medtronic Australasia Pty Ltd expressing concern about him purchasing the device online and encouraging him to see a neurologist.

I asked if Errol knew the 12 cranial nerves, baffling him with a little anatomy and physiology and the memorised list: 1 Olfactory, 2 Optic, 3 Oculomotor, 4 Trochlear, 5 Trigeminal, 6 Abducens, 7 Facial, 8 Vestibulocochlear, 9 Glossopharyngeal, 10 Vagus, 11 Accessory, and 12 Hypoglossal, asking did he want to risk damaging these nerves? Did he want, for example, his speech to be understood, to see and hear, talk, swallow, digest, and breathe adequately with a good heart rate, cough, sneeze, and smile? His sense of smell was already lost to Parkinson's. I was astounded at his medical arrogance and ignorance. I had already met a few people who thought they were God...One doctor I knew in another life, blatantly scribble-signed 'God' as his own name in a hospital register before surname printing became a legal requirement.

As Errol's speech was soft, pressured and very fast, many had difficulty understanding him. It was exhausting translating and keeping up with him. Many found it too hard and simply switched off. I also had to learn that he wasn't personally pressuring me when talking fast every day, as previously rushed snippy speech was because he was a bit annoyed. Now it seemed to me that he was always annoyed! So often, I just paused and took a few breaths, trying to concentrate as he ran everything out at a 100-mile-an-hour pace with few pauses and white froth around his mouth. I wanted him to speak for himself and was so pleased the speech therapists, encouraged him to speak with clarity and intent. Following the urgent tune-down of DBS, fortunately, he was stable for the visit by New Zealand nieces.

He was constantly looking for his job list which was written so small that it was illegible. Micrographia is another sign of P.D. It was exhausting for us both. I began to take over scribing for him and often had to interpret. We flew back from Asia to Brisbane, Australia for six monthly appointments, always keen for that sweet spot DBS setting without the mania, enabling him to function and feel tops. He knew it was there somewhere. I don't blame Errol for wanting the best he can get out of his DBS, who wouldn't? Medicos have a duty of care too. Parkinson's sucks.

Neurosciences Queensland some years later changed their telephone answering message. It no longer states they are the fifth best in the world for deep brain stimulation surgery. I mentioned this to Professor Silburn. His reply was, "We are now number three in the world," to which Errol very promptly retorted with a smile, "Well, I want to know, who is number one!" This is the kind of proactivity and dry humour that he has. He is straight to the point.

In Malaysia, Errol found a neurologist specialising in Deep Brain Stimulation and adjustments, making me extremely nervous. His settings were barely altered. I'm uncertain if they corresponded with Neurosciences Queensland. I had to be both on his side, wanting the best result and being his protector against that hot-wired setting that triggered disastrous mania, dissolving filters, increasing risk-taking and undermining stability. I had Skype set up for assistance for me if necessary. His proactivity in finding a better DBS setting extended to medics in Wisconsin, USA. He felt unimportant to the increasingly busy Brisbane team. He hadn't mentioned any USA travel ideas to anyone! Secrecy combined with impulsivity is concerning.

Quoting Errol, *"After an adjustment in Sept 2013, my whole life changed. Amazingly, I had an incredible amount of energy and had numerous projects going at the same time. You know 'leap tall buildings in a single bound' stuff. As a result of this extra energy, I seemed to have a falling out with just about everybody, it seemed they just couldn't keep up. Anyway, a further adjustment was done in late Sept. 2013 a virtual detune which slowed me up considerably, and I have been searching for the same energy without the side effects ever since."*

While I was in New Zealand during the Covid lockdown Errol began medical cannabis with an equal combination of Tetrahydrocannabinol (THC) and Cannabinoids (CBD). He didn't have pain nor suffer from the shakes, but it was a legal option for him to try, so he did. I returned to find him bright, slowed up and occasionally nodding off to sleep and hallucinating when visiting friends, plus physically 'plucking diamonds from the sky!' He also saw and spoke more with friendly ghosts aboard when awake, saying they spoke back to him. He insisted I talk with these deceased aunts, and a little girl one day. These visitations also happened before commencing Cannabis and blaming eye floaters didn't cut it with me. He had to agree, eye floaters don't have conversations! He has witnessed masses of insects crawling about the floors and also felt them on his head when off Cannabis. The 30ml containing 100mg/ml cost $180 so was also awfully expensive and should have interrupted normal driving. Perhaps he will revisit this therapy another time.

Nothing prepares us fully for life's major challenges, although we can learn and embrace them. Being proactive sparks change. I've learned that setting boundaries and priorities is important to balance my energies and enjoyment in life, staying focused on what else needs to be done or just needs to

199

be. Maintaining inner calm through loving vibrations, not fear, brings grace and ease.

Errol still is a doer and a go-getter, sometimes with great impulsivity. I especially love this aspect of him, but sometimes it drives me crazy as well if secretive. Communication is vital. Balance is critical. Safety first! We're grateful to have savoured such wonderful adventures at sea and continue navigating through life now in a reverse sea change mode as challenges dictate. We are setting up for security, safety and simplicity.

Quality sleep is important, snoring, snorting, and apnoea interfered. A priceless mouthguard resolved these. Every night, I never know if I will also cop a kick or fist thump while Errol's dreaming. He has a rapid eye movement sleep disorder. I worried about the presence of Lewy Bodies as these active dreams can be an indicator. There are many studies on Amyloid protein plaques in the brain causing the death of brain cells contributing to dementia. Alpha synucleins are indicative of Lewy Body Dementia. In time these tests will be more available with prophylaxis and treatment more specific. So far, Errol's low-resolution brain MRI has no alarming traits. I've gone through sleeping with my face protected and pillows between us. Whenever I lighten up, there's another dream surprise, helicopter arms, and a cry of, "Magpie- Magpie!" (swooping) for example. The latest was a lion and he roared at it, lashing out and simultaneously protecting himself.

Dreams often involved the police, sometimes he's fighting a croc, a dog, a deer, a snake, or some other demon that maybe just shot him! Occasionally, there's laughter and a jovial conversation to relay in the morning. Yes, it is a tad nerve-wracking for us both, and I learned to wake him also if snoring, check for his mouthguard, and reassure him where needed, avoiding a sore throat and maximising quality sleep. We do spoon. The antidepressants and melatonin made him sleep more soundly reducing active dreams as far as I recall. Improved medication is always welcomed.

His geriantologist backed the Souvenaid daily drink for memory. We attended the researcher's presentation of this product first. Red light and laser therapy are not endorsed by Neurosciences Queensland for DBS patients.

"Whether you think you can, or think you can't, you're probably right." - Henry Ford

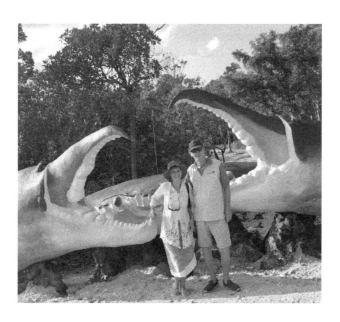

Recipe for a dream!

CHAPTER 12

ON THE ROAD AGAIN... IT'S GOOD TO BE ON THE ROAD AGAIN ♫

Northbound in 2014, after reprovisioning, we threw off the ropes and farewelled Runaway Bay, unaware we would cruise Southeast Asia for four years and return to Australia just before Covid. Taking time, anchoring along the Queensland coast awaiting the right weather to comfortably reach the tip of Cape York, cross the Gulf of Carpentaria to East Arnhemland, say Hello Yirrkala, continue through the gorgeous Wessel Islands, and eventually to Darwin. AHOY! These were well-beaten routes and hold happy memories. It's important to keep making the 'good ole days'!

✝ Royal Darwin Hospital offered some pool shifts. Feeling appreciated, I sharpened my skills, escorted patients interstate, adding new tools to my kit and a resuscitation backpack. Errol attended to boat maintenance. We enjoyed friends' company in the Northern Territory before crossing Joseph Bonaparte Gulf back to the generous richness of the Kimberly, W.A.

⚓ Reuniting with friends is always great. In Cattish Creek N.T., Les and Jill of MV Fiddler 5, and Robin and Reg of MV Catalyst welcomed us with a large shiny pot full of freshly cooked orange mud crabs on ice. Generously giving from the heart is priceless. Soon we were also 'mud-crabbed-out!' Whenever I think of mud crabs, this wonderful feeling of plenty and gratefulness fills my mind, even without eating them!

Fiddler 5's distressed guests meanwhile unblocked their flooded toilet, with us reassuring them that one day they would be busy catching barra in the Kimberley, laughing about it too!

Errol attended six-monthly neuro reviews in Brisbane, always hoping for adjustments to improve his DBS, medication and life. He seriously considered travelling to Wisconsin USA for the same. Sometimes, he calls himself a drowning man clutching at straws. Reduced mobility affected his ability to roll in bed. A silky bottom sheet helps. His feet still get sore from intermittent shuffling. His fast, soft speech deteriorated to the point where I often spoke on the VHF radio and translated for him, then a stutter developed. His very small handwriting had me attend to immediate paperwork (except online banking, which he resumed control over from family, after about 20 years of ease while we were away cruising Australia, to prove he could still manage it himself).

Relationships with his immediate family became more fragile. He had continued loss of smell, needed hearing aids, sixth nerve palsy gave him temporary double vision, his recall of treatment during the manic episode plagued his mind, sirens, even on TV, triggered his worst nightmare of admission to hospital against his will, and short-term memory loss was a new concern, intermittent festinating gait really added safety concerns. Some days balance is better. Letting go of control and accepting the loss of normal function added to feeling low-spirited. Errol also trialled adjusting his own medication looking for improvement. This did my head in as a nurse.

✚ Tips:

Consult experts. Get the team on the court with you; ask questions, share, and find a proactive neurologist, neurosurgeon, gerontologist, GP, physiotherapist, speech pathologist, dietician, dermatologist, ophthalmologist, occupational therapist, social and psychological advocates, friends, and family. Where families are distanced, busy or MIA (Missing In Action!) reach out and set up primary care and carer help.

Participate in healthcare. Educate yourself. Be patient. Learn about the condition and be safe, especially physically and with medications. Find assistance. Keep abreast of the latest breakthroughs and trials. Be open to new therapies. Join support groups when ready. Exercise. Eat healthy. Keep moving. Learn new skills, like cards, puzzles, languages, public speaking, crafts, instruments, cooking, boxing, etc. Have fun, practise cognitive exercises, meditation, yoga, or tai chi. Walk, swim, cycle, sing, dance. Do whatever and more of what makes you happy. Stay optimistic. Avoid stress. Help yourself. Help others.

Have a massage. Rest. Don't give up! Improve strength and balance and maintain independence and good social networks. Listen to your nurse; live your life! Start each day with a grateful heart. Sometimes we have to reprioritise and be open to learning lessons.

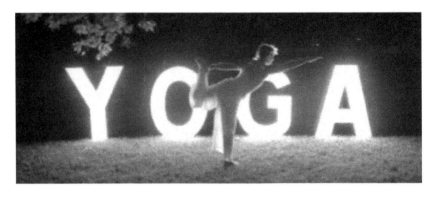

Yoga is life-balance.

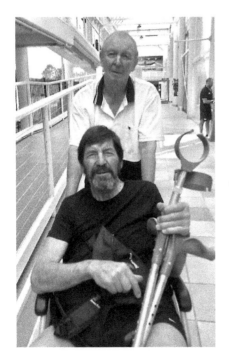

Errol and mate Mick Kowall (RIP) who also fuels my passion for a Parkinson's cure.

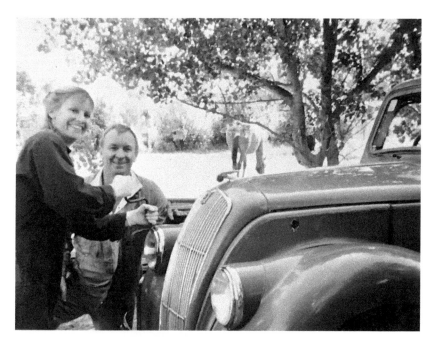

1939 Morris Eight. My first car (by default)
Errol's was an Austin A40

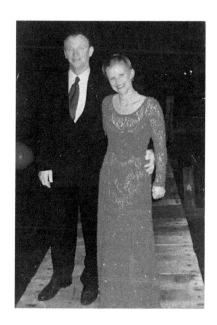

Walking the jetty at
Benoa Marina Bali.

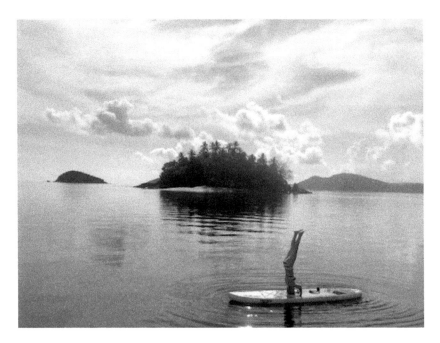

My goal was to headstand and I succeeded numerous times for long periods. As kids we had competitions to see who could stand on their head the longest. It's my thing!

We are grateful to Neurosciences Queensland for the ongoing support they give from their busy practice and from a carer's perspective, I'm aware it's wise to establish other helplines for the future, so we both have the best possible outcomes stepping into another chapter of our lives.

✝ The smile is the international language connecting people of all cultures and civilisations. It is contagious as naturally reciprocated, releasing dopamine. Muscle contraction has been shown a decade ago to be excellent for brain health, secreting stress-resilient myokines or 'Hope Molecules' (antidepressant-like hormones) into the bloodstream boosting mood. When we express appreciation, show recognition, give acknowledgment, and are grateful, the path to happiness lays out before us.

Remember the three C's in life...choices, chances and changes: and don't criticise, condemn, or complain. Sugar and salt may look alike but genuine sweetness is more palatable. Whilst I do practice mindfulness—enjoying each moment as it unravels—there are past experiences, learnings and baggage that we all have that make us who we are. Clearing guilt, fear, criticism and regret is bliss. It's sweet to romance down memory lane when the path is clear of any bad vibes. Some things we can be prepared for.

The decline in Errol's Parkinson's symptoms, fortunately, has been very gradual. Perhaps this was partially attributable to early treatment, proactivity, his 24/7 love nurse, and years of daily adventure, fishing, enjoyment and savouring wild-caught fresh fish loaded with omega three for healthy brains. Perhaps it's the hand dealt to him. Some days are diamonds, some days are stones. Yes, the progressive neurological degenerative nature of PD sucks. Everyone's journey is different, and every day has its own challenges. I hate seeing it slowly erode the man Errol was day by day, though actually, I don't notice it so much, as we are usually together 24/7. Being robbed of functionality is frustrating and it's amazing what he can do. Keeping busy doing what we love aboard was good therapy. I learned it's unnecessary to attend every argument I'm invited to, to choose my emotions, and to let my inner child play often.

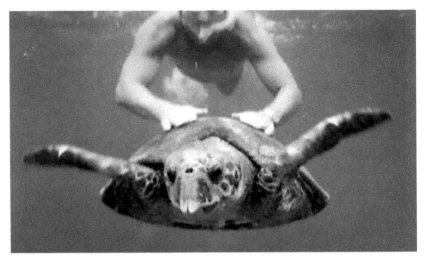

Green turtles are prevalent along the Queensland coast.

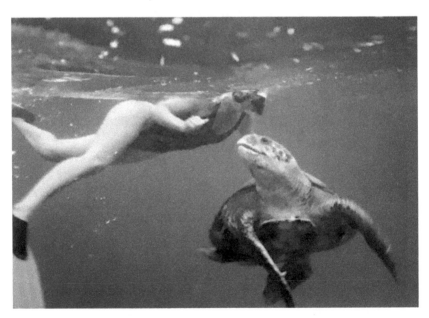

Turtles love pieces of fish and could easily take a fishy finger too.

Health care in Malaysia was world-class. Errol had a small Deep Brain Stimulator tune-up in Penang Island Hospital and follow-up scans of his chest in Kota Kinabalu once he survived a life-threatening bout of pneumonia (diagnosed and treated in Australia). The draining of a total of 3994ml fluid from his right lung really helped, as did oxygen and antibiotics. I stepped up to the plate, organising alternative boat care so I could fly to be with him and showed my unconditional love.

A recognised and concerning facet of Parkinson's is inherent vulnerability from the poorly functioning brain regulation centres, frontal and prefrontal cortex affecting executive functions in mood and behaviour, reasoning, problem-solving, impulsivity, gambling, and capacity for manipulation of emotions and finances by others (even imagined spousal infidelity) all with potential for crippling outcomes. Although a trusting soul, I've needed to be vigilant with Errol's spirit of generosity. Opportunists, keen to change their circumstances at another's expense, are anywhere in the world, including Asia and Australia.

We were taken advantage of, and an underworld of deception I'd not encountered in my fortunate life unfolded. We each make our own choices and our own beds and live with the consequences of our actions. I know in the past I've judged others for poor, illegal and immoral choices. Assisting subsistence locals with education and health fees was most acceptable, however, an Australian's Botox fee was not something I could support. Protecting Errol from those who subtly manipulate, endearing themselves to the point where he wanted to buy one a house; another, a guest's international tickets for an Australian wedding; especially since emotional manipulation, triangulation and deception was also evident there on a grand scale. The emotional toll was huge, and eventually, we both wised up to unwanted flying monkeys, theatrics and deception. Gofundme donations, charity and debit cards were for those in genuine need, not personal entitlement.

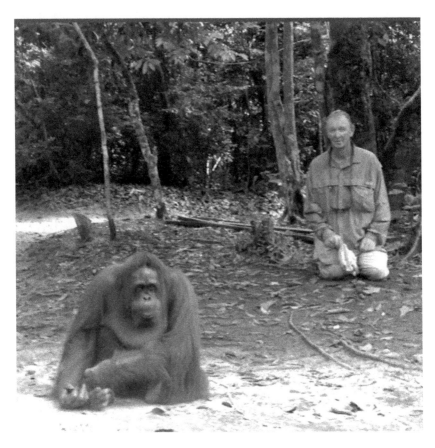

Siwa allows Errol to pose near Camp Leaky, Tanjung Puting Reserve, Central Borneo. We've helped out a few friends needing lifesaving antibiotics in Kalimantan for Typhus caused by Bacteria Rickettsia not Typhoid (Bacteria Salmonella). One friend Jenie Subaru of Kumai, with Scrub Typhus has affected valves and had worked closely with orangutans.

Manipulative people don't respect boundary concepts. They relentlessly pursue what they want, not caring about what or who gets hurt along the way. Lesson: let go of what no longer serves you!

Boat life can encounter a range of extreme situations. Our emergency injectable morphine supply was used recreationally by a professional (medical) friend of a friend, initially unknown to us, while aboard in the remote rugged Kimberley. This took a long time to piece together after discovering empty morphine boxes whilst routinely checking the expiry dates of medications when back in Darwin many months later, with some unaccepted explaining to the health authority who wouldn't renew our licence to carry controlled drugs. My character was not under scrutiny. Personal GP supply circumvented this bureaucratic red tape. Fortunately, I've never needed to administer injectable morphine aboard. We had utter disappointment in someone (now RIP) doing that to us at the expense of another's pain. Drug addicts must actively fight the demon.

Alone aboard in Thailand, while cleaning a cabin below, I found some chocolates, inadvertently self-overdosing, unaware that these three hearts were laced with drugs. My body is my temple. I wasn't happy. Fortunately, Errol returned, finding me drowsy and worried. Later, we were grateful I'd not taken a swim with an imaginary psychedelic turtle. Laugh if you like, but a child could have found them under the bed, I could have died and our boat could've been confiscated.

We had someone holding a steak knife to their own throat.

Another aspect of Parkinson's is emotional instability. It's vital that travellers on a boat are mentally sound. Someone who puts themselves, the boat, or others at risk is a real threat and can cause potential disaster. A captain must be able to recognise where these risks exist and act upon them swiftly, recruiting professional support. The lessons that we learned, impacted by Parkinson's, were to have open communication, be alert to manipulators, trust gut instincts, and have strong boundaries in place. Expect nothing and be prepared for everything!

Letting go of what no longer serves us and offering forgiveness is self-care. Letting go of those who deceptively poison the soul gives the ultimate respect to our own relationship with healing, forgiveness and freedom. We are all an evolving work in progress. Grace and truth are free gifts of richness.

Keeping healthy aboard is imperative. It has been an extremely rare thing in all our years of voyaging for me to ask anyone to improve their performance as a team member. We're easy-going and know that no one likes to be criticised, even if constructive. Most people are very considerate of others and our home when aboard. A happy, balanced, cohesive crew is important for the smooth running of the ship.

In my early days aboard, the need to entertain and keep others occupied seemed more necessary, often as a sea-sickness distraction. I've learned to slow the doing and just 'be' more. There is always plenty to do and see. Closely monitoring water usage, as boaties do, was reduced by our fabulously generous desalination plant, and it was a joy to share fresh water, ice, and our big washing machine.

Our fabulous, adventurous world-cycling French duo, helped with whatever they could, staying welcome aboard for five months instead of just one week for the Sabang Marine Festival on small Wei Island just North of Sumatra Island, Indonesia. Free travel, board and food, made it a win-win for all our guests.

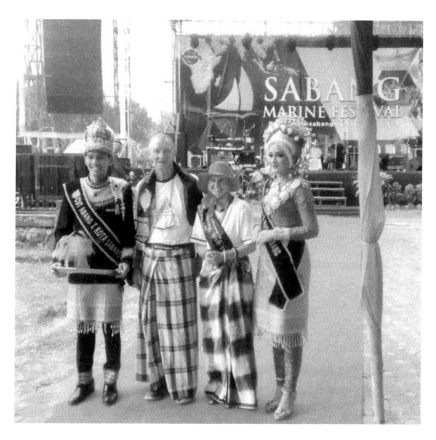

Sabang is in Aceh province, at the northern tip of Sumatra Island. Here I also learned some Arabic.

Different backgrounds make us who we are. Recognising and appreciating strengths builds self-esteem. It's hard being anxious when grateful. When we have food, shelter, something to do, someone to love, and something to hope for, we have every reason to enjoy life.

"Try to leave this world a little better than you found it, and when your turn comes to die, you can die happy in feeling that at any rate you have not wasted your time but have done your best." — Lord Baden Powell

Lord Baden Powell also said, *"The most worthwhile thing is to try to put happiness into the lives of others."*

⚓ Some occasions call for action before words. There are good and bad people everywhere. Safety aboard is paramount. Here are some of our pirate stories; I hope these may also be a page-turner to world peace, beginning with the golden rule: treating others as we wish to be treated and each of us loving one another.

The Malaysian and Indonesian Governments have zero tolerance for pirates and drug runners. Some are also identified as terrorists.

*Trained Abu Sayyaf decapitators rob, kidnap, and kill for money for their own cause. They will hack off your arm or head, rape, and plunder without a second thought. They also get killed. We were shown such photographs by the Malaysian police as reassurance before going around Borneo's tip.

*North Borneo, South Sulu Sea with heavy Malaysian flotilla security, our seven-crew shared two-hourly night watches, practiced mock under-attack action plans, from known active South Philippine pirates, locking ourselves in our engine room and biding time for East Sabah Security Command rescue. The extinguisher, glucose, VHF radio, torch, phones, etc., were ready.

*South Philippines, a South African skipper we know directed a flare into a pirate's fast runabout once alongside following up with a Molotov cocktail. Boom! If carrying weapons, you must be prepared to use them without hesitation or you're dead meat first.

*We decided our prepared Molotovs were a danger to ourselves and we'd likely be shot first. None of us knew if we had the courage needed to survive such an attack.

*One Japanese sailor's spouse followed in her husband's footsteps once he was knocked unconscious, giving such a loud fight for her life that the kidnappers left them alone cut, pistol whipped, bleeding, and unconscious as she undoubtedly would have been too much trouble for them ashore.

*Remember Kiwi round the world yachtsman Captain/Sir Peter Blake, defending himself, was fatally shot by pirates who stole an outboard motor and watches from the crew. RIP.

*German Hendrike Dielen of SY Catherine shared her six-month kidnap trauma in Jolo South Philipines by Islamic Abu Sayyaf Militants. Eventually, she agreed to befriend one of her captors making time a little easier. Her husband was tortured, kept in a hole he dug and threatened with decapitation. Millions were exchanged. Most governments refuse to pay blackmail ransom.

*Robbed at Blupblup Island, Papua New Guinea (PNG) when ashore, a village elder paddled dugout asking, "Someting E miss? Sansoose!" pointing at our feet. Much more from outside and our shoes were stolen. He returned what he could.

* An opportunist invited us ashore at Manus Island, PNG, then robbed us. Entering through the upstairs wheelhouse window, he exited with saloon-level goods via the same window, not using downstairs doors! He transported items via dugout canoe to the uninhabited island's plantation, covering them before a rainstorm. The rainbow alerted me to the missing camera and more. A huge amount of gear was recovered. There was shame in being caught. Errol threatened to chop off the thief's fingers with our bush knife, frightening him.

*We returned to Australia, then had an outboard and fuel tank stolen from the dinghy while reprovisioning at Shute Harbour. We weren't happy rowing the long way back out to the boat with the load. There are many beautiful and peaceful places to be in the world without drama and fear. It all starts from within.

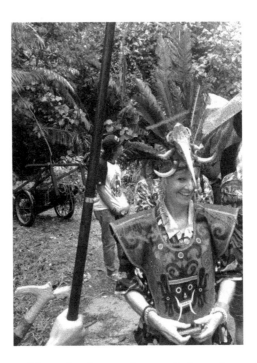

Preparing to blow the (non poisonous) dart through the pipe bursting balloons with Dyak tribe, West Kalimantan, Indonesia.

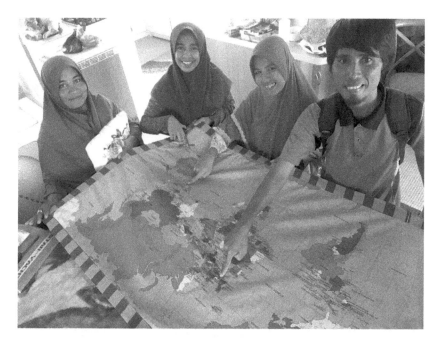

School teacher Wahyu Di Udin from coastal Kilo, West Nusa Tengarra Indonesia, travelled to Norway. He organises beach clean ups and teaches youth to be clean and green, and is very inspirational and enterprising. Bismillah and Alhamdulilah! Before everything, give thanks and praise. Hallelujah!

May our homes be blessed, and peaceful havens oozing love from every corner. When stepping beyond the roadblock, will I first ask permission or beg for forgiveness? Do we forgive ourselves and others or hold resentment? Are we true, kind and considerate? Do we let the ugly in others kill the beauty in ourselves?

I believe confronting resistance is a powerful barrier buster that may show up uninvited in many forms; as the truth (sometimes naked and hurtful), an ogre with a heart of gold, a long-lost friend or foe, a stranger, an untimely visitor, an opportunity, a welcomed surprise or gift, a long hug, possibly invisible, as freedom, courage, faith, a guiding light, a random act or word of kindness, questioning our own core beliefs, our integrity, our care factor and our compassion, with boundaries, or a resolution, as a pearl of wisdom, as a need for understanding, as another hidden way, and for closure.

To these ends and more, I'm happy to enthusiastically share the bright life of Claire White, Claire-Light, Claire de Lune, Claire-Voyant, and sentient, savouring the love joy, and hope of midwife 'sage femme' wise woman. Happy is my playful inner child. I am resilient and can get through anything. I am enough. I've dropped the act of being everything to everyone.

I shine and can light-up others. I have the power to calmly change direction slipping into the ease of the ebb flow, instead of battling against the current, to love, nourish and heal, reflect and reassess myself and treasure my life's journey.

😇 When we let our love and light shine, we're, in a sense, a lighthouse: strong and powerful, able to bring some safety, security, solace and sparkle to others, and at the same time, allow our own inner light to shine a little brighter. This empowers all to connect to feel-good hormones. These, in turn, set up the circuit for continued connection, clarity and cheer. We learn to ride that wave of life force, feeling exuberance and joy in amazing balance with magical confidence that comes from knowing the choice is ours. Action is power! Jive into the dopamine dance of life, swim in the oxytocin ocean of love, sleep in the serotonin serenity lake of the living, stand energised on that wave riding on endorphins, and may a tide of loving inspiration wash over us lifting us up to our full potential.

♥ Having the gift of the gab, Errol has always joked that my life's allocated quota of words could run out mid-sentence! Of course, he refers to talking not writing, but I can let my words flow out bravely. Kindness matters. With respect, it's the basis of the golden rule.

With maturity, we learn to set boundaries, goals and priorities, knowing others can feel disappointed or upset, knowing we manage our own feelings, and don't have to go to the default yes response; I can speak and stand up for myself. Reality check: no matter what I do, say, or write, or what I don't, despite being respectful and all-inclusive, I acknowledge that it is what it is. A carer needs caring too.

"You can please some of the people all of the time, you can please some of the people some of the time, but you can't please all of the people all of the time." John Lydgate

---

May you find your completeness! We usually only get one shot at this life, so make it a joyful time well spent. May your true colours sparkle and shine. Smile and love each other. We learn along our journey. I'm grateful also for the beautiful gems that just drop into my lap. I choose compassion, trust, wisdom, truth, joy, light and love. My Claire cup is full and my fountain of small talk flowing.

I hope reading this breathes extra life into you and that you, in turn, breathe it into others with added love. Keeping our individual cup so full it's overflowing is important, and only allowing others to drink from the saucer, prevents depletion and keeps our outlook one of abundance. I love life and it loves me.

I appreciate Errol and the opportunities he has given us all by being bold, brave, and kind, a hero and an impulsive legend. I intend to faithfully remain his magnet for miracles, loyal and lovingly looking to the future, focusing on the good and people who treat us right, keeping us light with unconditional love, knowing the more optimistic the perspective, the more worthwhile and enjoyable the ride.

Get clear about what you want in life, consider new evidence-based strategies for understanding challenges and ways to process resistance and rigidity, calming the nervous system. Do the action needed to get out of the dark. Face fear and let it go. Unravel the mind rewiring with more compassion, reducing struggles letting in light and love, illuminating pathways with our own sparkle to bring healing and peace. Raise energy to bliss.

"I'm sorry, please forgive me and thank you, I love you..." May the power of this ancient Hawaiian Ho'opnopono prayer of forgiveness also reach your heart and soul, bringing unity and an unbreakable bond connecting us to everyone else, even though we seem so separate, allowing reprogramming of the subconscious mind for better healing. Amen...and so it is.

May you find strength, courage, composure and compassion.

"May the long time sun shine upon you, all love surround you, and the pure light within you guide your way on."
Mike Herron

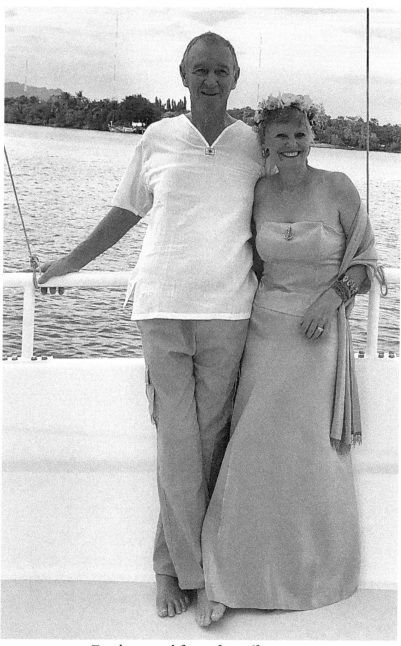

*Footloose and fancy free off we go to
another wedding- in Thailand.*

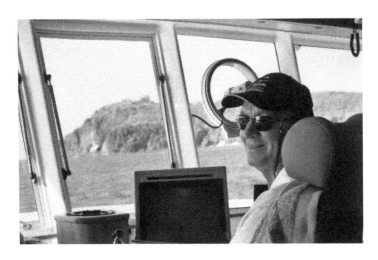

*Passing Double Is Point happy to be in
charge and homeward bound.*

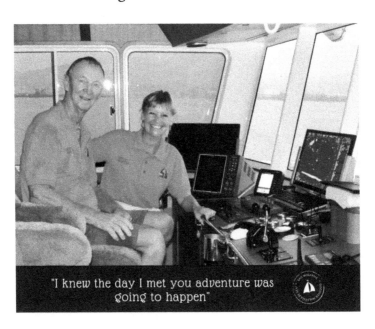

"I knew the day I met you adventure was
going to happen"

*Yes! Wildly amazing adventures! We continue with enthusiasm,
optimism and courage. I pray for kind hearts, fierce minds,
brave spirits and that his physicality continues to defy
medico's negative expectations with thanks until the end.*

The Man in the Arena.

It is not the critic who counts, not the man who points out how the strong man stumbles or where the doer of deeds could have done them better. The credit belongs to the man who is actually in the arena, whose face is marred by dust and sweat and blood; who strives valiantly, who errs, and comes short again and again because there is no effort without error and shortcoming; but who does actually strive to do the deeds; who knows the great enthusiasms, the great devotions; who spends himself in a worthy cause; who at the best knows, in the end, the triumph of high achievement, and who at the worst, if he fails, at least fails while daring greatly, so that his place shall never be with those cold and timid souls who know neither victory nor defeat.

—Theodore Roosevelt, April 23rd, 1910.

Again, I thank you for contributing to Parkinson's Research through purchasing my book.

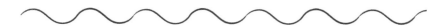

ABOUT THE AUTHOR

Claire was born near Southbridge, a farming community in Canterbury on the South Island of New Zealand. Large influencers in her life are a happy, loving family, helping others, guiding, the great outdoors, music, travel, languages and especially the water. Introduced to other cultures at a young age, she has a unique, adventurous, and quirky free spirit.

She became a New Zealand registered general and obstetric nurse (RGON), consolidated training, then returned to French Polynesia, nursing in an exotic cosmetic surgery clinic. Tropical life, ukulele, guitar, and drum music with Polynesian singing and dancing, international cruising yachts and magnificent sunsets grounded and inspired her.

Midwifery, family planning, hyperbaric nursing, radio operator, advanced diver, and Australian Citizenship certificates were awarded in Darwin, Northern Territory, Australia. She also learned to sail and windsurf there, loving accident and emergency work. Her mental health first aid and palliative care certificates were completed in Queensland.

Before the internet age, she travelled around the world for 10 months, attending a Hyperbaric Medicine World Symposium and Conference in Washington D.C. and Boston, U.S.A. From Cairns, Queensland, Australia, she set off sailing her first Coral Sea Classic International Yacht Race to Papua New Guinea's Port Moresby, winning line honours and becoming hooked.

From Darwin, she crossed the Arafura Sea, winning line honours on her second International Darwin to Ambon Yacht Race to Indonesia, competing annually until joining her husband Errol with race radio communications including a Tall Ships race in the Madura Sea. Meeting her adventurous life partner, pilot, and captain Errol at the Darwin Sailing Club was a dream come true. Together they have made a life few dare dream of cruising for decades aboard 80' Restless M with her history of treasure hunting, drug running and pirates.

Claire loves life, people, and nature and oozes positivity. A Queen's Guide Award recipient, she formed her own Girl Guide Company and learned to fly in Derby, Western Australia. In Darwin, Northern Territory, she led Malak Brownies. She continues to collect and play many musical instruments, enjoying adventure, and exploring the great outdoors.

She hostessed aboard Pionair's DC3, flying all over New Zealand. Delivering babies of friends and family and palliative nursing humbles her to the sacred, fragile and miraculous cycle of life. She has a natural fun-loving, joie de vivre and sparkle.

Cruising full time for nearly 30 years, especially in Australia's remote Kimberley, Oceania and Southeast Asia, despite her husband's Parkinson's Disease diagnosis at age 56, she used her nursing skills especially when balance became a safety issue aboard, then reverse sea changed to a land-based home at Hope Island on the Gold Coast.

Claire is also a qualified yoga instructor, teaches ukulele, and is a force for good, knowing her worth. She is passionate about helping others better understand Parkinson's, fundraising for research for a cure, and is grateful for your contribution. She believes she can, so she does!

Claire's contact details are:
Email: idlewise@hotmail.com
Whatsapp: +61456805648
Website: www.clairewhitespeaker.com

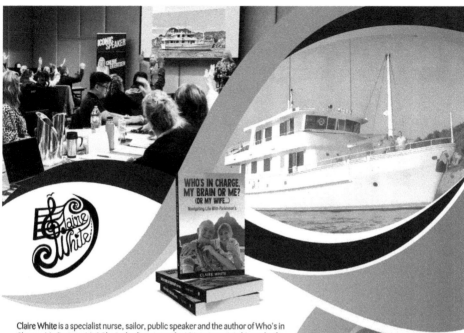

Claire White is a specialist nurse, sailor, public speaker and the author of Who's in Charge, My Brain or Me? She is the first mate of a 180-tonne mini ship and wife of Captain Errol was diagnosed in 2002 with Parkinson's disease over 21 years ago. Having lived a unique lifestyle on the water for almost 30 years, Claire is passionate about raising awareness and funds for research and a cure.

Helping others better understand their individual concerns inspires Claire. Her extraordinary personal story of living with Parkinson's aboard demonstrates the joy in living the dream life of adventure with compassion, empathy and hope.

Her expertise is invaluable and her cheerful, open, and grateful heart is evident in everything she does despite facing a reverse sea change and becoming land-based. Claire remains dedicated, motivated, enthusiastic and passionate about making a difference in the world starting at home.

Parkinson's Disease – Remaining Resourceful

- Unpacking symptoms and complications
- Psychological and emotional strategies for a quality life
- Problem-solving on the go…

The Cycle of Life and Its Colourful Beauty

- The heroes on our journey
- Support is everywhere
- Dealing with grief and celebrating life

Cruising off into the Sunset

- Discover what floats your boat
- The beauty and mystery of our World
- Sustainable practices for the longevity of our planet and ourselves.

Contact details: 📞 +61456 805 648 ✉ idlewise@hotmail.com

ACKNOWLEDGEMENTS

Firstly thanks to God: Bismillah.

Errol, you've shared the challenges, and supported and guided me into my birth as an Author. You are The amazing star, and I love you, unconditionally as I love family.

This book has been possible also through perseverance and the patience of some very good friends who gladly gave hearty encouragement and advice. You know who you are. I give you thanks.

Some thank you's are in the text, some not. I'm grateful to all who've helped us, especially Ian and Cathy Aylward, the entire team at Ultimate 48 Hour Author; Natasa and Stuart Denman, Julie, Vivian, Lendy, Wendy, Rebecca, Nik and Velin. Friends Julie Fickel, Kerry, & PJ Mancini especially your techie help made the difference and saved my sanity. Others have shared their expertise in various ways.

Many authors have influenced my life, Jaishree; I look forward to travelling with you and sharing our stories. Iconic Speaker family you have boosted my confidence, JT Foxx you blow my branded socks, off the block, and Kaley Chu's entire positive team of influencers is outstanding.

To my wee group of 'Ukulele Sistars' for keeping me sane, allowing me to gaily offload whilst topping up my cup, you really went up and over. Joy, Jacquie, Jenni, Linda, Leanne, and Dianna, Maree, Julie and Cathy thanks. Laughter is the best medicine and music sings to the soul. A shout-out to my Halcyon community for acceptance and understanding of my slowness to become involved until this book was done! Now here's to you the reader for coming on this journey around the world with us, for being forgiving and generously contributing to raising funds for a cure. Three cheers for you in health, wealth and happiness.

TESTIMONIALS

I have known Claire White for nearly 30 years. In that time, I have watched her go through the extenuating circumstances of nursing and supporting her husband Errol through the debilitating disease of Parkinson's.

She has faced each challenge 'head on' with the deep love of a wife and the professionalism of the experienced RN that she is. I have seen her at the worst and best points of her journey. She has been tolerant and compliant when needed and her morality is beyond reproach at all times.

If Claire has a fault, it's her total selflessness during the very challenging times of dealing with this incurable illness and the challenging effects on her and her husband.

I commend Claire most highly.

Nanette Clifton
Author of *The Muddier the Water the Brighter the Blooms*

Navigating seas and oceans is daunting for anyone, let alone someone with Parkinson's Disease. PD affects the brain's control centre, impacting movement, thinking and mood.

I have known Claire, a dear friend for 40 years, and Errol for 28 years. We shared some truly amazing adventures: Darwin to Ambon yacht races, the Arung Samudra in 1995, the Tall Ships race in the Madura Sea and cruising the Thousand Islands. Living on their beautiful boat was pure joy.

Extraordinary oceanic adventures, yacht races, and dealing with pirates are now no longer on the radar.

Do yourself a favour and enjoy this wonderful true story that takes you on an amazing journey, providing great insights into a travelling boat life, our brains, living with Parkinson's Disease, Deep Brain Stimulation, stem cell and other treatments, special friendships and so much more.

Claire's kind heart and soul captured Captain Errol's heart and together they have lived life to the fullest with many adventures and much laughter, sharing beautiful sunrises and sunsets. This is their life journey.

Debra Ann Curran
RN Darwin; Midwifery QVMC Melb; FPWNP
Darwin/ Adelaide; Grad.Dip.Spec.Ed Melb Uni;
M.ED(Hons) Melb Uni; M.MCHN Latrobe Uni

Claire has an incredible memory and she has an amazing story to tell.

I have known Claire (and Captain Errol) for almost two decades, working as midwives together whenever she returned to Gold Coast, QLD. There's an exquisite, alluring joy that Claire carries, camouflaging and transforming her own struggles and challenges with Errol.

Their story is incredible. Claire's faithful devotion to Errol during their adventures on the high seas, while navigating the dark waters of Parkinson's, is evident on every page.

This is a testimony to her patience through the stormy challenges of tuning-up hyperdrive, frequent falls, medical appointments, and life on a boat. It's an insightful, authentic account of living with someone with Parkinson's.

This book offers hope to the newly diagnosed and their families, with empathy and consolation to those already on the journey.

Enjoy.

Julie Fickel
Dip Nursing
Grad Cert Health Science Midwifery
Post Grad Dip Mid
Dip Art and Counselling

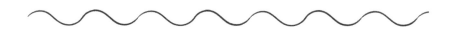

NOTES